Aloha

The Message of Hawai'i

Anolia Orfrecio Facun

Chelsea Tyson   Leslie Tyson

All Scripture quotations are taken from The New King James Version/
Thomas Nelson Publishers, Nashville: Thomas Nelson Publishers. All
rights reserved.

What A Wonderful World Publishing titles are available at special
quantity discounts for bulk purchases for educational, business,
fundraising or sales promotional use.

ISBN: 978-0-9846405-0-8
Library of Congress Control Number: 2011924754

Published by What A Wonderful World Publishing

95-2031 Waikalani Place D601 Mililani - Honolulu, HI 967689
(808) 294-4499
or online at www.ECKOBooks.com/product/1002146/Aloha/

Printed in the United States of America.

Dedication

To all of the wonderful people of Hawai'i
who breathe and live the Aloha spirit

Acknowledgement

To *the People of Hawai'i*, thank you for sharing your beautiful islands and the message of "Aloha!" to the rest of the world.

To the mother-daughter team, *Leslie & Chelsea Tyson*, whose dedication to the preservation of the Aloha and wellness shared among the people of Hawai'i, gave me enough inspiration to create this book and help accomplish such a dream to be possible. Completing this project became a reality because of their tireless effort.

To *Victor*, my dear husband, whom I call the "Aloha boy" for his love of the island and the people, and for his great support to this Aloha project.

To everyone who contributed to make this project possible - Our writer contributors who generously shared their time and writing abilities through their stories: Honolulu Mayor Peter Carlisle, Kahilinai McCarthy, Pastor Wayne Cordeiro, Teresa Shuptrine, Sylvia Dolena, Dalani Tanahy, Holan Nakata, Gloria Cohen, Cheryl Toyofuku, Lee Miller Lane, Dr. Charlie Sonido and the Bayanihan Clinic Without Walls Team, and Constantine Nightingdale who also helped us with the glossary of terms; Erika Taylor Montgomery for spending lots of hours doing her expert editing and Pauline G. Cabansagan for some as well; to our Community Partners, Sponsors and Contributors who supported our mission, and to all other participants who gladly volunteered and shared our efforts to make a difference in our communities, our deepest appreciation. Also to the Hawai'i Visitors & Convention Bureau for providing some needed information and resources. Our great appreciation extends to Stephanie Robertson of Ecko House Publishing who served as our wonderful Publishing Coordinator, Dustin Kritzer for the beautiful cover design, Amy S. Catlin Wozniak for publicity and marketing support, Nathan McCotter and countless individuals who extended their Aloha spirit to make this project possible. Mahalo! We can all say, "We did it!" and together, we can continue to make a difference in people's lives with the beautiful message and spirit of Aloha.

Contents

Introduction

"Aloha!" From the time anyone starts to make plans to visit the world famous tropical Hawai'i Islands, there's that great feeling of joy, picturing one's self being welcomed by the beautiful sunny weather, blue sky, fresh air, fresh fruits, relaxing around the crystal clear water, beautiful leis, watching or dancing hula with the Hawaiian dancers in grass skirts, and on and on. Yes, I'm one of the visitors who keep coming back. Yes! I've got to admit, my husband and I LOVE HAWAI'I! Catching the Aloha spirit of the island, we wish to make it someday our home.

We have visited Hawai'i as tourists four times, two from winning a company's contests, one for a business leaders' incentive with another company, and the last, a cruise out of curiosity of what the other islands look like. The cover designs of my books were taken from the islands of Hawai'i.

Now, I'm going deeper into the mysteries of Hawai'i. The island is not only beautiful with those mentioned tourist attractions we normally associate the island with. There's definitely much more than those... I'm intrigued, challenged to say the least, to find out more.

Herein, you'll find contributed stories, anecdotes, a bit of history, and some helpful information when you come to visit Hawai'i, from contributing local Hawaiian writers gracious to share their experiences, love and care though Aloha.

Most of all, in the end, we hope for both residents and guests alike, that you'll rekindle your love and appreciation for this "home" which most visitors will work a month extra or put their entire year's savings up to visit. As we share the wonders of the islands, let us all collaborate in an effort to preserve the message and spirit in Hawai'i, the land of ALOHA!

OFFICE OF THE MAYOR

CITY AND COUNTY OF HONOLULU
530 SOUTH KING STREET, ROOM 300 • HONOLULU, HAWAII 96813
PHONE: (808) 768-4141 • FAX: (808) 768-4242 • E-MAIL: mayor@honolulu.gov

PETER B. CARLISLE
MAYOR

DOUGLAS S. CHIN
MANAGING DIRECTOR

MESSAGE FROM MAYOR PETER B. CARLISLE

It gives me great pleasure to offer my perspective on **aloha** for the book: Aloha the Message of Hawaii.

The name of our island, Oahu, also known as "the gathering place," belies the importance and meaning of our way of life. It is our tradition of aloha that unites immigrants, visitors, locals and native Hawaiians and promotes the sharing of ideas, cultures, and traditions.

Our island is a special place—a sanctuary of *alii*, kings, and queens—where leadership passes through generations and imbues us with hopes and dreams and the energy for innovation, collaboration, and productivity. The way of aloha is demonstrated through our celebrations and gatherings which incorporate family values, *pono*, and honors the past while looking towards a sustainable future.

While aloha can mean both hello and goodbye, it is not simply a word, but a tradition of graciousness that binds our community together. It is the thread that runs through a lei and holds the constituent elements together to form a whole.

It is because of the allure of this tradition, unique to the world, as countless others past and present have done, I chose Oahu as my home, to work, live, and raise a family. On behalf of the people of the City and County of Honolulu, I share our warmest aloha to all who enjoy this unique spirit and tradition.

Peter B. Carlisle

Peter B. Carlisle

3

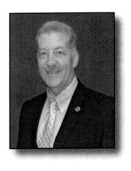

Peter B. Carlisle is serving in his first term as Mayor of the City and County of Honolulu. He was elected in September 2010 to serve as Honolulu's 13th mayor. Carlisle was born and raised in New Jersey and came to Honolulu in 1978 after receiving his law degree at UCLA. He began his career as a Deputy Prosecuting Attorney for the City and County of Honolulu shortly after his arrival. In 1989, Carlisle was employed as a partner at the law firm of Shim, Tam, Kirimitsu, Kitamura, & Chang.

In 1996 Carlisle ran a successful campaign for Honolulu Prosecuting Attorney and was re-elected four times over the span of 14 years. He successfully tried such notable cases as the Xerox mass-murder which resulted in a life sentence for Byran Uyesugi.

Carlisle's administration as prosecutor is distinguished for its political independence and advocacy for common sense in the justice system, where among other things, he along with the law enforcement community, successfully pushed to implement Information Charging which created a more efficient way to initiate felony cases.

During Carlisle's administration, Honolulu experienced historically low crime rates which he credits to inter-agency cooperation and collaboration efforts.

Carlisle met his wife Judy and raised his daughter Aspen and son Benson here in Honolulu.

The Search for "The Message of Hawai'i"

Anolia Orfrecio Facun

It was September 2010, and I was contemplating what's happening in our world today - what I refer to as the gloom and doom feeling in the environment - when I suddenly thought of Hawai'i. I remembered the beautiful feelings I had whenever my husband and I visited the islands. As a tourist then, we mostly stayed in Waikiki and did not miss the round-the-island tour in Oahu. Nature lovers like us appreciated the natural beauty of the island. It seemed like such a small space, but there was so much to see and everything was so delightful to look at – the almost always blue sky with constantly moving various types of clouds; the mist of rain that occasionally came by to refresh us and the land; the huge, beautiful rainbow, sometimes multiple, that constantly pop up right before your eyes; the turtles, whales, dolphins and other sea creatures abundant in the Hawaiian waters; gorgeous flowers, delicious fruits, etc. The list of things to admire and behold in your heart is endless.

But there's more... Our experiences while watching the Hawaiian people who are always kind, hospitable, friendly and helpful. During one of our tours, I remember the guide saying that "Everyone here are cousins." As we visited the not-so-tourist areas, and as we got to meet and befriend some people around the islands, we noted the closeness in both immediate and extended families. It is true, families gather just about every weekend in the public parks and beaches having barbeques or parties and such. They looked vibrantly and genuinely happy! Yes, that's what I was looking for when I went back to Hawai'i, to find out more about this special trait of the Hawaiians, the strong sense of family and community values.

One time we were invited to a huge family get-together at the beach. The Bantolina family has nine children and all together, with their spouses, children and grandchildren, total of over fifty members in just one family. We will never forget the warmth in our hearts when we were told that we are now also a part of their family. It is such a wonderful feeling that we have a "family" to call in Hawai'i, a family to visit whenever we come. This must be the Aloha.

Also at that time, the wonderful Williams family, introduced by a local friend, had a spare room in their home and welcomed us to use it instead of a hotel for our longer stays. Being with them reinforced to me the values you sometimes miss in busier communities: hospitality, friendship, caring and sharing are just a few of the remarkable traits still alive and well in Hawai'i. Truly, besides the sense of fun and entertainment, I feel the world can learn a lot more from the island of Hawai'i.

So what is the message of Hawai'i?

Whenever we visit Hawai'i, we book flights with our favorite airline, *Hawaiian Airlines*, of course. You surely feel the vacation as soon as you embark the plane – the greetings, the friendly stewardesses in uniform, the special movies to give you a preview of the island experience, and the magazines which I read from cover to cover (there's plenty of time). I am determined to know everything I can about Hawai'i.

This fifth visit was definitely different from the others. I did not come as a tourist, but I wanted to experience being one of the residents here. I will not deny that the thought of just staying here, and making Hawai'i our home came to mind. Our friend Maria was again gracious to share a room in their home. I was so

7

grateful. My husband was not with me on this one-and-a-half month trip, so I had to drive myself around the island. I brought funds to buy a simple used car. But then, what was I to do with it if or when I had to go back to California? Renting a car would be very expensive. The biggest challenge is driving around the island. I found it difficult to be familiar with the street names; they all seemed to look and sound the same. Guess what? I decided to experience the island's public transportation system which I'd heard is very efficient.

The Bus

Yes, for over a month, I took and made transfers on The Bus, its actual name. I loved it! I got to meet many people. All types of people in Hawai'i use The Bus, which is mostly full, sometimes standing room only - many students, professionals, market shoppers, service officers, tourists, and sometimes homeless people. It's a warm feeling to see that our elders and folks on wheelchairs are able to go around town with peace of mind. They are well cared for, with seats reserved for them right at the front section of The Bus. The drivers are always ready to assist while the buses are all equipped with ways and means to make life easier for everybody, very efficient without unnecessary delays. I smiled thinking, "how thoughtful of the management." The youth are also oriented to give seats to the elders or women in need. This natural care and preserved values are so refreshing to still observe. I learned a lot and had many great experiences to remember whenever I took The Bus. Those trips made up some of the most memorable moments in my life.

I lined up my activities, places to visit and events to attend based on whatever I could find in the island paper, the *Honolulu Star Advertiser*, my "what, when and where" buddy. I practically read each copy from cover to cover and it was a great help. I had it all planned out. I was on a mission to search for "the message of Hawai'i."

Kalihi

My first visit was to an annual event in downtown Honolulu, called the *"Kalihi."* Bands were playing, great singers took their turns, dancers of all ages performed traditional and modern dances, and there was simply a general sense of family and community. I was very impressed with the sixty four year old lady who still gracefully and energetically danced both traditional and modern hula. She also teaches youth of all ages to dance hula. This is another thing I love about Hawai'i: it doesn't matter what your age, size, shape or form is, anyone and everyone who likes to dance is welcome to dance hula! I truly enjoyed that day. Even though I was alone, you can never really feel alone because everyone there is so friendly and helpful, like they've been your neighbors. There was a lot of food, arts and crafts to purchase, and many service booths to learn about valuable community resources. I had so much fun and learned a lot. This was an excellent community event. I am already set to join the next one.

Hawai'i Five' O

My next stop was the *Hawai'i Five' O Premier* event, at five in the afternoon at Sunset on the Beach. I was so glad I was taking the bus. The entire Waikiki Beach was packed that day, so it would have been nearly impossible to find a parking space if I had a car. You could feel the excitement in the air. Hawai'i Five 'O was a very popular TV series back in the '70s. I talked to several young and old fans from all over the place already crowding the beach early to be part of this comeback celebration. WOW! The band that had been playing beautiful Hawaiian and other familiar music suddenly went silent, then the most familiar Hawai'i Five 'O background music filled the air. The song was welcomed by a huge cheer from adoring fans and the crowd sharing that special moment with the new cast of this sure-to-be hit TV show. There were bikinis, bare chests and legs, endless food, beer, music and colorful outfits, commemorative t-shirts and cameras flashing everywhere. It was an exciting moment! Noticed or not, it was a peaceful day when people from all over the nation, or world, gathered in one place like one big family just having fun and having a party! Big thanks to Hawai'i Five 'O for the great shows and wonderful memories. I love the Aloha way!

Princess Kaiulani

A post from a known bookstore caught my attention: The cast for the movie, Princess Kaiulani would be at the store that Saturday afternoon. My young friend Chris would bring me there. I was naïve. I had never heard of the movie or the name of the princess. It surely interested me though to hear a bit of Hawaiian history. I went, and found it even more interesting that the back area of the bookstore for such gathering was packed; all seats were taken. This must be a popular movie, I thought.

The directors and producer were there besides some cast members. I remained standing till almost the end. There were great discussions, followed by more questions and answers. Then I realized that those present were not only absorbed by the movie portrayal of the characters, but the actual history and the emotions involved in the takeover process of the Hawaiian monarchy remained fresh in some of the people's hearts. I have to admit that at that moment I knew nothing about the island's history except it was once under a monarchy until it became America's fiftieth state. That's it. It was a quick decision then for me to determine I needed to know more about how that happened. After mainly just listening to everybody speaking and sharing their praise, disapproval or opinion, suddenly I found myself raising my hands before they closed the session. I said, "I've been listening and keep hearing this 'message of Hawai'i,' which is the reason why I am revisiting the island. Who is the best person to tell me more about this movie you have?" Before I knew it, I had an appointment to interview the producer and the directors three days later. I thought, "I don't know what to expect, but this is becoming more interesting."

On my way home, still thinking about my experience at the bookstore and my upcoming interview with the producer and director, I realized I didn't have any tools for that. I only had with me a small digital camera. I felt a mild panic. How could I face these professional movie folks and interview them with a small digital camera with recorder? I immediately called my local friend Nenette for rescue. Fortunately, she knew of a video guy that I could possibly call. Benjie, his name, was too busy and not available at all to meet with me to discuss details prior. But he was kind, and learning more of my predicament, agreed to meet with me that morning to shoot the interview. How could this be possible? I never met this man, had no preparation, had never been to the Princess Iolani Palace or had any idea where it was in downtown Honolulu. That morning, it was a bit of a disaster due to the fact that in a rush to get to the place so I would not be late, and wondering if the man to help me would actually be there, I left my prepared interview questionnaire in my room. In the end, it turned out to be a miracle because a brand new friend, Leslie, was kind enough to volunteer to bring me to the Palace, and there, with all his equipment in hand, was Benjie! That was a memorable day. In Hawai'i, I felt you never had to feel alone or like a stranger. You never realize how many friends you actually have who can pull off such miracles! Was I discovering the Aloha of the land? That day keeps my heart warm with a smile whenever it comes to mind.

The way I did the interview may have not been the best it could have been, but I surely learned a lot from the experience and I was awakened with the gained knowledge of Hawai'i's background. I thanked the producer and directors of the Princess Kaiulani movie for instilling the awareness in me. For me, especially in these present days, this was not just about a very interesting Hawaiian history of a royal monarchy who had lost their throne or kingdom. Involved here are people, special people who struggle to keep on in this land that used to be their own, and a very special culture struggling to stay alive in the islands of Hawai'i.

I still have so much to learn, about the past, the present and what the future will bring to this paradise land. So, where do I go next? What is the message of Hawai'i?

Back to The Bus

I made frequent visits to Chinatown to buy various kinds of delightful food and any other interesting things I can find. My favorites were fresh fruits, young coconut, boiled sticky corn and peanuts.

One day, I apparently got onto the wrong bus. The bus was moving on and at first I didn't know what to do. I supposed I would not get lost in such a small island, right? Somehow, I exclaimed with a smile to the lady next to me, "I'm on the wrong bus!" She smiled back and told me not to worry. Julie assured me she would get me to the right bus so I could reach my destination. I felt a sigh of relief. I thought she would just tell me what to do next. No, she stopped the bus, insisted on walking with me across the street for about a block, and made sure that I got on the right bus with full instructions on what to do next before she left to go her way. I was amazed! How nice and beautiful she was to do all that, taking her time to make sure I would really be all right. That is ALOHA! The more I experienced living life in Hawai'i, the more I knew this was the place I would love to be. I began to realize that I was not only finding "the message of Hawai'i," but I was also finding a "home."

Just Give Me Hope

Another memorable moment I had while riding the bus was that one day at the bus stop waiting shed. It was a beautiful day and I was really enjoying the clear blue sky and great weather. I noted four people there, a woman and three gentlemen, quietly waiting for their bus to arrive. As I approached, I said to everyone, "Good morning!" They acknowledged my presence, but no one said anything. I thought that to be strange. And then, I got this look like, "That's weird that this lady is talking to total strangers." The woman smiled a bit so I sat next to her, and continued talking to my new friends, mentioning how beautiful it was that day. I noted the man at the end of the bench, who, by his appearance, may possibly have been homeless. I couldn't help but notice his long locked hair, about to his waist. I was curious so I asked, "Would you mind if I ask if that hair is real?" He simply nodded, without a word. I continued my conversation with the folks there, whether they replied or not. They appeared to be listening and being attentive though. Then I noted the man with long hair beginning to tap his two hands on his lap. At first softly, then progressing to a more rhythmic motion. Then suddenly I heard him singing! He had a beautiful voice, and the hymn sounded good. If only I could understand the lyrics. Then, as he seemed to be getting carried away by his song, I began to distinguish some words: "Just give me hope, give me HOPE." We were all quiet once again, watching what was happening and listening to this man singing.

But then, two buses, one after the other pulled over. He got up to go on one while I was going to the other one. As we crossed paths and we were at same spot, I paused and told him, "I heard you singing. You have a beautiful voice. I hope I will meet you again someday so I can hear your song." As he stepped onto the bus, he gave me a beautiful gentle smile. I will never forget that day. It was like something happened in that bus stop, with that man, and possibly with everyone else who was there who heard and witnessed the man singing that beautiful song. We all got separated inside, but as I tried to find the people who were with us at the bus stop, I spotted them one by one, interestingly looking at me also. They seemed to lighten up, with more life and even a trace of smile in their faces. I knew there was that special joy that stirred in my heart that day. Did we, too, catch more hope for the day? If we could only share more HOPE and LOVE in this world, we would always be assured of VICTORY in life! Could this be the Aloha spirit I was catching, and sharing with other wonderful folks of the island?

Then it hit me. YES! That's the message of Hawai'i... the ALOHA, in the full meaning of the word. Aloha is definitely not just hello and good-bye. It is a lot more than that.

Ten days prior to my scheduled flight back to the mainland, my husband followed to spend time with me on the island. It was time for me to go home and he was making sure. We enjoyed the rest of those ten days together, almost like how the tourists do it, except I wasn't feeling like a vacationer anymore. I felt Hawai'i was where I really belonged, as I began to tell my husband my adventures on Oahu Island. I had him take the bus with me on occasion while I shared my stories and how much I loved it here. He could see my excitement, my joy. I gained a better understanding of Aloha each day. This time not just knowing of the word, but I was actually feeling and living Aloha!

Changes are Happening in Hawai'i

I have to admit that what I observed in Hawai'i during my last trip was not all beautiful or pleasant. Since I have been going back and forth a lot now between the island and mainland, it is possible that the changes I am noticing are more pronounced. It somehow bothers me that there are now too many homeless people all over the place – parks, streets, bus stops -everywhere. Some not too touristy areas by the beach were lined with tents and makeshift huts for the homeless. Not that they bother me or I mind them, but I was sad that there are so many homeless folks and I feel many are not living in a dignified way as human beings. Why is this happening? By the way, during my last visit in January 2011, after a bill was passed concerning the homeless situation, I noted that the makeshift camps disappeared. The beaches are all cleaned up, but where did the homeless go?

It also became noticeable that there were more and more modern stores around. So-called "progress" is everywhere now, to the obvious resistance of some residents. It's evident by the huge signs in front of their houses expressing their disapproval of the welcomed changes.

The changes among the children are more visible as well. Instead of the happy conversations I used to see among students gathering or walking everywhere, I now see with them what I used to see only in the mainland: tied up with their cell phones or headsets. It used to delight me to see the younger generation walking hand-in-hand, talking or teasing each other, giggling or laughing, doing usual youth stuff. Now I noticed that sights like these are much diminished due to their newfound preoccupation with their new modern gadgets. The truth is I am missing the sights I used to see. I can't help but feel some sadness, and maybe a feeling of being alarmed, that Hawai'i's youth are catching up with indifferences that are becoming common among the youth of modern cities in the mainland, sometimes bringing depression and isolation. Now you can't help but wonder... Is this what you call "progress" or should we be more aware of some danger signs?

As a community health advocate, I can sense these symptoms don't belong in the place of Aloha. I hope the adults and youth alike recognize these signs and symptoms while it is still early, and do something about them. The beautiful people and families don't deserve to suffer the consequences brought by commercialism that only benefit the merchandisers more than the consumers. Not all gadgets are needed or helpful. Especially on this island where people used to be very happy just by being with their family or friends without any of the modern stuff that now occupies them. They are not aware that these new things are keeping them away from their family and friends whom they love, their source of support, real security and joy. What can be done?

The Message of Aloha Project

The beautiful lady I mentioned earlier, named Leslie, has a virtual assistance business, which I believe is possibly what I may need to assist me while travelling back and forth between the mainland and Hawai'i. She has a beautiful daughter named Chelsea who is in high school, and is currently being homeschooled. As I watched these two ladies together with their closeness, the mother-daughter relationship, and how they share and work together in many aspects of life – schooling, church, daily life demands and even political conversation, I developed a respect and admiration of them, and a sense of responsibility. How do we preserve this type of lifestyle here in Hawai'i? I had a conversation with the two of them. How about if we put together a book that aims to help preserve the Aloha in the islands?

A book project was born to seek out more of the true meaning of Aloha; to share and remind our "Ohanas" to continuously make an effort to preserve this beautiful and valuable part of Hawaiian culture. Thoughts also came that we hope we can raise some funds to help celebrate our youth's talents and potential, and to help bring back the dignity and opportunity to the homeless citizens of the island. These are the shared desires of the few with whom I had a chance to share what was burning in my heart. This project would take a lot of time and dedicated effort. But with Leslie and Chelsea making the commitment and being excited to help, it was possible. They would be my co-authors. The decision was made to go for it. It would be much better than not giving it a try or do nothing.

So it happened. We share the determination to preserve the Aloha in our beautiful islands, not just in our thoughts but in positive action. We cannot allow Aloha to fade or die. What will happen to these beautiful islands if our future generations lose the very essence of Aloha that keeps Hawai'i the way it really is? She is beautiful, because her people are naturally beautiful, inside and out.

Aloha, the Message of Hawai'i

First, I learned the other way of writing and saying "Hawai'i" with the apostrophe symbol in between the two "i" letters. Second, since I am a new resident and still absorbing all I can about the island's culture, I thought it would be best if we allowed the locals to be contributors to the book. We invited recommended locals from different backgrounds to provide written contributions on a voluntary basis, to narrate what for them is the meaning and message of Aloha. We had several great community leaders and members who enthusiastically responded and liked the idea. We were very encouraged by this expression of support. Within two months, I was reading the first submitted drafts Leslie provided. I thought I was just going to read a manuscript. Instead, I suddenly found myself in tears, tears of joy. I was overcome by the writers' expressions of Aloha, like the overflowing joy I feel when I see a bright rainbow, which reminds me of God's love and promises. Yes, there is hope, there is a way, Aloha for the islands of Hawai'i is here to stay! To our locals, my wish is that may you revisit and rediscover our precious Aloha. May you find more meaning and truly value living a naturally good life in Hawaiian culture, a life full of Aloha!

And to all our visitors and guests, my hope is that next time you visit Hawai'i, you treat yourself to something beyond the obvious. Experience the spirit of true ALOHA. Mahalo!

****

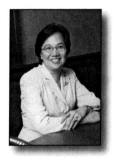 **Anolia Orfrecio Facun** is an active Community Health Advocate and the Bestselling author of the books *Yes! The Secrets Work!* - Discover Your Unlimited Potential and Purpose in Life; *Game Changers* - The World's Leading Entrepreneurs, How They're Changing The Game & You Can Too, and several more. Anolia is a lady with a mission: To share and show people, regardless of circumstances, how *abundance* can actually be achieved by simply understanding and applying "Total Wellness" principles. For over thirty years, Anolia dealt with and witnessed thousands of people go through life's complexities in search of happiness, health and prosperity; and drew conclusions based on life's basic principles, science, logic and simple common sense. These basic human principles are nothing new, and still apply: People need wellness in all areas of their lives to experience *completeness* or *total well-being* and its naturally occurring abundant result.

Anolia is also a public educator, social entrepreneur, community volunteer and avid traveler. She was born in the Philippines and came to America at the tender age of twenty two as a nurse, with a suitcase and a few dollars in hand. She knew nobody nor had an address to go home to when she arrived, although she was asked to report to work the day following her arrival. Her experience as a young recruited nurse in this new land of America was a story by itself. She managed to cope, survive and even thrive through all the learning experiences she went through. Thinking of how these experiences and valuable lessons learned over thirty years would all just go to waste if not passed on, she decided to put them in writing and share through her books. In all these, she acknowledges God to be her ultimate source for everything. You may find her books on Amazon and BookFinders.com

She recently founded what has now become the "Total Wellness = Abundance" project with the purpose of reaching out to individuals, businesses, and communities to go back to the *basic human principles* in dealing with, or managing, their daily personal, career, business or social lives. It works! To learn more about Anolia, her works and mission, and/or how she can share with your group, visit www.YesTheSecretsWork. com. She will gladly help.

The Seaweed IS Always Greener... in Hawai'i

Chelsea Tyson

As soon as I started high school, it suddenly hit me.
College was coming up, and it was coming fast! I had
entered the final stretch of school before I would be
off to college. Even though I was excited, the thought
also made me anxious because I only had four years to
sort through thousands of colleges and pick just one!
I was clueless as to what my "top 3" or even "top 10"
choices were, but I had made my mind up about one
thing concerning college – it would definitely NOT be
in Hawai'i.

Like Ariel in *The Little Mermaid*, I thought everything
is so much better, easier, and bigger in the "mainland."
As her little crustacean friend Sebastian said, I thought,
"The seaweed is always greener in somebody else's lake."

I just could not see myself getting great opportunities here on this "small, secluded" island. To sum it all up, I couldn't see myself "making it big" here in Hawai'i. Now, with college now only a year and a half away, the decision of whether or not I will leave for college or stay here, is becoming harder and harder to make.

My view of Hawai'i has changed immensely in the past two years. Although I can't deny that Hawai'i is obviously smaller in size than the mainland, the opportunities here are far greater than I initially thought, and one unique aspect of Hawai'i, I found, is the root of all the opportunity. When I really contemplated it, I came to the conclusion that the only way a small island can have such big opportunities is because of ALOHA.

To me, "aloha" is so much more than a greeting or salutation; it is the attitude of the people here. Because there is a spirit of aloha deep in our island's foundation, we are all one big Ohana (family). When you think of it this way, compare it to a big, loving family. Sometimes we get along, and sometimes we don't, but most importantly, you can always rely on each other to be there for you and support whatever ambitions you have. In fact, because there is a feeling of Ohana in Hawai'i, the fact that the island is small actually contributes to it. You see, when you have a small family and someone makes even the littlest achievement, it does not go unnoticed — that's how it is in Hawai'i. When you set forth to do something great, you not only have a whole island behind you, but, when you succeed, it does not go unnoticed and, in a way, it brings us all together. If you don't succeed, they still "got yo' back" and encourage you to move forward.

Aloha is what brings us together in good times and in bad. I know that sounds cliché but it is so true in Hawai'i. I know this state has seen its share of ups and downs, just like I have seen mine, but thankfully, we both are blessed with a big family that pulls together and can pull through anything that comes our way.

I still don't know what college I will be going to in a little over a year, but I will not go back to my prior view of Hawai'i. No matter where life may take me, I will always be proud to call Hawai'i my home!

****

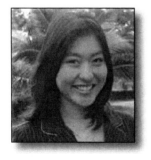

Chelsea Ayano Tanaka Tyson is a 17 year-old world traveler with an expansive personality, an active life style, and an exciting dream for her future. She lives "smack dab in the middle of the island of Oahu, Hawai'i" with her parents, Morris and Leslie.

She seldom sits still as her favorite activities include hiking, tennis, and running. Chelsea's need for excitement bubbles to the surface in the form of her all time favorite activity: travel. Since her birth on April 17, 1994, she has traveled to Japan nine times and to India once.

Chelsea is an only child, but her family is not small. Though none of them live with her, two step-brothers, one step-sister, and one half-sister all make up Chelsea's family. Two indispensable members of the Tyson family are a bunny named Bijoux, and a finch who wishes to remain anonymous. Two other things Chelsea could not live without include watermelon and ice cream.

Not only is Chelsea a traveler, she is also a thinker. This is her third year as a homeschooler—officially a junior at the high school level. The best advice Chelsea says she ever received is, "Don't live in the past, or you might miss out on the future." And her future surely looks bright. Chelsea dreams of becoming a journalist—first, as one who travels around the world, then, as a work-from-home freelance journalist. These are some pretty ambitious goals, but she believes she can do it. Just as her favorite Bible verse says, "The Lord will fight for you; you need only to be still."

Ua Mau ke Ea o ka ʻĀina i ka Pono

The life of the land is perpetuated by righteousness.

- Hawaiʻi State Motto

Aloha, A Way of Life

Kahilinai McCarthy

When I was so graciously asked by Leslie Tyson if I could share my thoughts (mana'o) on what the word "aloha" meant to me I was honored. And I thought that it would be easy for me to put it on paper. It was not! As I thought of the word "aloha", tears started to well up in me. I started thinking about how much "aloha" is a way of life. It is the foundation, I believe, for and in the Hawaiian culture. But aloha extends from and through all the people of Hawai'i. I was fortunate to be raised in the Hawaiian culture, where my family lived "aloha" daily. Aloha is an extension of love, loyalty, kindness of the heart, a willingness to welcome others into your presence and extending an invitation to share with other's your heart. Alo, means to be in each other's presence, as we greet one another. Ha, the breath, which

I refer to "life". It is a greeting which is a "way of life". We live "aloha" through our lifestyle, our attitudes, our beliefs, our spirit, and our acts of kindness, which overflows to the world.

There are many stories I could share about living in the "land of Aloha". So many people of Hawai'i taught me that "aloha is a way of life." But it would take me writing a whole book. So allow me to share one of the most heartfelt stories of "aloha" that I experienced.

I was fortunate and blessed to have been a part of Aloha Airlines for 34 years, before Aloha's final closure. I grew up with Aloha Airlines. I worked alongside the most wonderful people, who through the years taught me the deep meaning of a word we can sometimes just say, and not mean. The "aloha" that comes from a sense of belonging was so very evident at Aloha Airlines. Aloha Airlines was known as TPA, before it was renamed Aloha. People referred to TPA as "the people's airline." And of course, this was before my time. Yet, the spirit of "the people's airline," TPA, extended well into the airline soon to be renamed Aloha Airlines.

It was the year 2005, when I was diagnosed with breast cancer and had to go into treatment, which meant I would not be working. I was then a single mother with two daughters. Since my treatment would extend over a period of five months, and recovery another few months, I would exhaust my vacation and sick leave. My fellow flight attendants donated thirteen months of their vacation time for me. As I write this, I cannot contain my tears. For you see, Aloha Airlines was in bankruptcy and all employees had to take a twenty percent pay cut. But that did not matter. What mattered was love, trust, friendship and loyalty. They also created an "Aloha meals on wheels," and brought dinner and groceries to me and my children for five months. An Aloha pilot would purchase a wig for me without my knowledge, and other pilots would deliver groceries as well. Aloha... a way of life, I know it first hand, demonstrated by people who lived it. The people of Aloha Airlines, because aloha mattered.

Because we live in Hawai'i, we sometimes take the hospitality and values of the Hawaiian culture for granted. But I believe there is a need for us, as an island people, to intentionally live "aloha." It is not only for us, but for those who come to Hawai'i, with such great expectations of the "land of aloha." And it is a privilege for us to be able to extend this gift we have to the world. We, at Aloha Airlines, were honored to be given that privilege for over sixty six years. Aloha never ends, because it lives in the heart of everyone who embraces "the breath of life."

Aloha... a way of life.

****

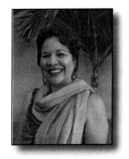

Kahilinai McCarthy was born and grew up in Honolulu most of her life. In her younger years she also lived in Los Angeles, San Francisco and Richmond, California.

Kahilinai attended many different schools as she was growing up living between California and Honolulu. Eventually her family settled in Pearl City, Hawai'i. She attended and graduated from Waipahu High School. Pearl City High did not exist yet.

She attended Leeward Community College for two years, then started her long thirty year career with Aloha Airlines in 1974, as a flight attendant and in-flight instructor. Her career at Aloha Airlines also encompassed being an "Ambassador of Aloha," traveling to many different countries, promoting Aloha Airlines and the Hawaiian Islands. After Aloha closed, she then went to help with the start of Mokulele Airlines and became their Director of Customer Service.

Kahilinai traveled extensively throughout the world in her first fifteen years with Aloha. Married in 1987 to Michael McCarthy, she had three daughters, Kalei'i, baby Na'i (deceased) and Melissa (affectionately known as HoneyBee).

She now has two grandsons, Noah and Oliver Begley, whom she adores.

She also has her own business in the health industry, Juice Plus. Her business came about when she went through breast cancer, and learned the importance of nutrition.

Kahalinai has been a member of New Hope Christian Fellowship since 1996, and is presently active with the Prayer Ministry and Market Place Leadership.

An Uncommon Aloha

Wayne Cordeiro

Aloha is a simple but profound word. It may be as simple as a child's hug or like an elderly couple walking hand-in-hand, silhouetted by a rich sunset, it can hold a lifetime of meaning.

It is used for a greeting or a farewell. Much like the Hebrew word, *le cheim* which can be interpreted, "Life to you," Aloha has much to do with life!

It also has to do much with love, but a quality of love that supersedes what we hear in most romantic songs or see on the silver screens. This kind of quality can be discovered in these islands, if you look closely enough to find it.

As beautiful as the beaches are in Hawai'i, that is not our greatest asset. Neither are the undulating mountains of the Ko'olaus or the gently swaying palms that dance before the white sands of Haleiwa. As prized as these beloved ornaments are to Hawai'i, these simply frame something far more compelling and attractive.

It is the *love and respect for the life* found within these islands that bring us together to enjoy the landscape and scenery that has inspired hundreds of compositions over the years. The fresh breath of life has always been so precious to those who live in Hawai'i. The ancients would stand *face-to-face*, and there breathe on each other as a blessing and a way to communicate the deepest meaning of love.

Each weekend, you will find tents and umbrellas pitched before sunrise to mark a spot for ohana to gather, and here we find an example of the essence of aloha. No, not simply the gathering of families, but the life found teeming within them ... the laughter, chatter, and the banter. It's discovered within the stories that are told and retold as memories come alive around hibachis and BBQ's. Whether it's at the Ala Moana Beach Park or under the many canopies that line the beaches of Waimanalo, the life of aloha can be found.

For me, *aloha* holds even a deeper meaning.

I have become an avid student of the history of Hawai'i as far back as King Kamehameha I. His wife, Queen Kaahumanu, was the primary ali'i that banished the kapu system in 1819. Shortly after that, missionaries from the New England states, prompted by Henry Opukahaia, arrived on the shores of Kona. Shortly thereafter, the High Chiefess Kapiolani, Keopuloani and other citizens became devoted Christians.

A new era had begun for Hawai'i.

The ensuing years would spin the tapestry of Hawai'i's history. Missionaries, kings and queens, sandalwood, and whaling all made for a slow but steady transformation. This Pacific Paradise brought together colonies of Chinese, Portuguese, and Japanese as they came in boatloads from far-flung countries. Today, the eclectic mix of who we are is a result of that intermingling along the way, the beauty of a human alchemy of precious people who are grateful for who they are, where they came from, and what they have become.

However, our aloha for one another did not come without a price.

One unique characteristic that sets Hawai'i's people apart from many other countries is that we live on islands confined within the borders of our Pacific Ocean. In earlier days, navigating the seas was not as easy as it is with today's air travel and ocean liners. People were compelled to live with one another, accept one another, and at times, tolerate one another. And when the toleration levels were exceeded, battles to solve the disagreement ended with bloodshed and lost lives.

Then when the spears were still and the musket powder finally subsided, aloha had a chance to once again appear. Aloha cannot grow in discord. It can only thrive in peace. Since 1782 when the whalers arrived, wars, battles, the struggle for land, pineapple, sandalwood, and power punctuated the chronicle of our islands' history. As radiant as Hawai'i's aloha is, it stuttered and stammered under the stewardship of men and rulers, captains and conquerors.

Here is where aloha holds a deeper meaning for me.

I grew up in the Palolo Valley, a tropical embrace at the foot of the Ko'olaus drenched in greenery and blossoms of the plumeria and hibiscus. My mom, a single mother, worked as a waitress at a local restaurant and raised me and three other siblings. Our surroundings were sparse but we lived aloha. We developed a palate for tripe because it was the cheapest commodity my mother could buy. (Tripe is the lining of the first or second stomach of a cow.) But it went down easily and our opu's were full because we loved each other and our ohana was all we had.

But then came the worst of times. Despite all her efforts, my mother could no longer afford to raise her batch of children, so our divorced parents agreed to split the family. Two of her children went with my father and two stayed behind with mom. My brother and I were sent to Japan to live with my father who was in the Army. Within a week, I was separated from everything I knew and held dear. After three years, we moved to the West Coast of North America.

It was during my second year in high school when the worst took place. For months, mother, who continued to reside in Honolulu, wrote successive letter asking that I return home. Although only in her 40's, my mother's kidneys had failed and in those days, dialysis machines were scarce. Five people needed the treatment using the only machine the hospital had, and my mother was not one of the chosen to receive treatment until another machine arrived.

I asked my father to send me back to Hawai'i, but he refused. Two more months passed. It was during my math class. A telegram arrived and was hand delivered notifying me that my mother had passed away.

I remember running from the classroom with the crumpled telegram in my hand. Finding a tree in the school's garden, I began pounding my fist into the hard bark until my knuckles bled. My anger for my father and for God simmered. And like the early Hawaiians whose toleration levels were exceeded, I defiantly left home after threatening my father. A year passed, and I dropped out of my senior year in high school. I finished my education through a correspondence course, enough to get me enrolled at a community college known for its jazz program.

It would be there in the Pacific Northwest, that I would find the meaning of Aloha.

Campus Crusade, a Christian collegiate organization, sponsored outreach events sharing the Gospel message and came to my town. One particular evening I found out that they would feature a music group. Being a lover of music and an avid guitar player, I attended the crusade. It was here that I heard the invitation to again revisit the One whom I had turned away from, the One the Bible called the God of Love. I still blamed Him for the untimely death of my mother, and my heart was closed to anything that had to do with such an uncaring god. However, the zealous disciples of Campus Crusade were persistent and I was invited to other group gatherings and outings. Hearing the Gospel message of God's love again and again made me hungry to know more of this God who cared.

Slowly, my frozen heart began to melt, and over a period of a few months, I knew that God was love and not hate. He was merciful and not angry. He had a bright future for me if I were willing to accept it.

The etymology of the word "Aloha" is actually the combination of two words. "Alo" may mean, *in the presence of*, and "ha" is the word for *life*. So Aloha can mean: *to be in the presence of life*.

There is no greater blessing to anyone than speaking aloha to a person …to be in the presence of life!

Finding God's love brought me there.

I look back now over 36 years ago, and discovering God's aloha brought the most significant change ever.

Man's love, when tested and challenged, will erupt into war. God's love, when tested and challenged, will heal you and change you.

I am still learning about the unending meaning and application of aloha, but finding God's love has made my heart teachable again. That in itself is one of the most beautiful things of the word we may never find the full meaning of until we see Him face-to-face, and He breathes on us the deepest meaning of …

Aloha.

****

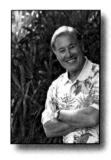

Wayne Cordeiro is the founding pastor of New Hope Christian Fellowship in Honolulu, Hawai'i with over 14,500 in weekend attendance. New Hope is also listed as one of the top ten most innovative churches in America with Outreach Magazine listing them as one of the "top five churches to learn from." New Hope is known for redeeming the arts and technology. Over 3000 attending services each week via the Internet. New Hope has seen over 73,000 first time decisions in Hawai'i since its inception 26 years ago.

Wayne is a church planter at heart with over 108 churches planted in the Pacific Rim countries of the Philippines, Japan, Australia and Myanmar. Nationally, he has planted churches in Hawai'i, California, Montana, Washington, and Nevada.

He has recently accepted the role as President over his alma mater, Eugene Bible College, recently renamed New Hope Christian College. NHCC is now part of a consortium of Pacific Rim Christian Colleges with locations in Hawai'i, Oregon, Myanmar, and Tokyo.

He has authored ten books, including such classics as *Doing Church as a Team, Dream Releasers, Seven Rules of Success, Attitudes That Attract Success, Divine Mentor, Leading on Empty* and to be released soon, *The Encore Church.* Wayne is also the author of the *Life Journal*, which is being used by thousands of churches worldwide, is bringing people back to the Word of God.

Pastor Wayne and his wife, Anna, have three married children and four grandchildren. His hobbies include music, reading, water sports, and riding his Harley Davidson. Wayne and Anna now split their time between Hawai'i and Eugene, Oregon where they have a family farm. There he leads New Hope Christian College, writes, and enjoys spending time with his grandchildren.

CONTACT:

Wayne Cordeiro c/o Mary Waialeale, Admin. Asst.

290 Sand Island Access Rd.   Honolulu, HI 96819

Ph. (808) 842-4242 ext. 113   Fax (808) 842-4241

'A'ohe lokomaika'i i nele i ke pān'i

No kind deed has ever lacked its reward.
An opportunity to help another is a gift.
To live with Aloha is to have a giving nature.
Give for the pleasure of giving.
Do not expect something in return.

A Bowl of Aloha

Teresa Shuptrine

Out in the yard we were ever so blessed to have a thriving gardenia bush. It was almost difficult to keep up with the fresh multitude of morning blossoms that arrived overnight. The smell was thick and sweet— almost intoxicating!

It was a family affair. Every morning, "Uncle" would bring in an armload full of blossoms and put them in the sink. My sister had the painstaking task of washing and removing the tiniest gnats that would bury themselves happily in each bud. The blossoms were bundled with love and presented to me daily.

I had the privilege of quietly praying each morning after seeing the harvest and asking the Lord who to bless with the flowers that particular day. I would immediately get several names of people who would receive the elegant prized buds. I would head off to work and enjoy the task of placing a bundle on the desk of the recipients of the day.

It often brought smiles to weary faces in the morning. Each one would light up as they eagerly grabbed the highly fragrant flowers and brought them to their noses. I so enjoyed delivering and watching their expressions. It was similar to the satisfaction of smelling a delicious cup of fresh brewed coffee, I thought — differing aromas that would stimulate and awaken your every sense.

As I prayed one particular morning, I got just one name. Then I prompted the Lord, inquiring, "Who else?" Silence. This had never happened before! I told my sister and she went into the closet and got a big, beautiful etched glass bowl that she ever so carefully wrapped and handed to me.

I drove to work puzzled that morning. As I entered the office I went to Joannie's office. She has one of the most stressful jobs any human could possibly endure. She heads a unit that investigates children that have allegedly been physically, emotionally, and sexually abused or neglected. I felt so honored to be chosen to present Joannie with the "gift."

My heart sank as I was told she would not be in. I questioned myself for a moment — but a knowing is a knowing. I put the huge array of gardenias in the beautiful bowl with water and lovingly placed it on her desk in her office. As I walked past the office window and looked in, I was amazed at the elegance of the flowers in the bowl. The staff asked if I wanted to leave a message. "Tell her it's a bowl of *aloha* from God."

I went about my business that day. Returning to the office late in the day, I was met by my boss. She was pacing back and forth and yelled when she saw me. "Where were you? The phones have been ringing off the hook - Joannie's been looking for you!" Knowing me, she added, "And what have you been up to now!?"

I anxiously went to Joannie's office and was met with a huge smile and a bear hug. She ushered me into her office and she could barely speak. As I peered at the bowl between us, it seemed as though the buds had exploded into enormous blossoms—it caught my breath!

Joannie began to slowly speak as the tears filled her eyes. Along with the daily stress of the job, she had gone to the doctor that day and received bad news. She paused for quite a while, trying to compose herself.

"Whenever I'm down," she said, "I go to Chinatown and get myself a gardenia, because it always cheers me up. Today, I went to every flower shop in Chinatown and could not find one gardenia! I was devastated, as this had never happened. I became even more depressed than ever. I forced myself to go back to work and you could not imagine my shock when I laid eyes on the massive bowl of gardenias on my desk! The room was so heavenly fragranced — I sat there crying, as they told me 'It's a bowl of aloha from God.' You are truly a heavenly messenger," she said.

"Yes," I said, "but it's all about the message…"

****

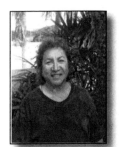

Theresa Shuptrine was raised in Haleiwa, North Shore of Oahu. Naturally caring, she worked with physically and mentally challenged, blind or visually impaired children, incarcerated youth, child protected services, recruited and served foster families. She also parented special needs foster children.

Theresa's philosophy and passion: "To love and serve others," which is her way of sharing the good news. She likes to help empower others to fulfill their destiny, by seeking and using their gifts and talents, to be all that they can be for themselves and others. She wants her (achievements) ceiling to be the floor for others, meaning, she wants her highest accomplishments to be their base standard.

Theresa is an inspiration and a blessing for many lives she is able to touch. She is determined to live her purpose driven life towards a purpose accomplished life.

Aloha, the Divine Breath

Sylvia Dolena

"Aloha, to learn what is not said, to see what cannot be seen and to know the unknowable."

~ Queen Liliʻuokalani

I would never presume to speak to the experience of Hawaiians. Being Native American though, I can certainly identify with aspects of their struggle, loss of precious land, suppression of language and culture and I certainly empathize. Through it all the *real* Hawaiians maintain the Aloha spirit, with reverence for the land, ocean, even vegetation and animals. I dedicate this story to them, the real heroes of this land of Aloha, the divine breath of life.

I live on the Big Island of Hawai'i close to the ocean and ridiculously close to the volcano. After visiting Hawai'i in 1986, I always expected to live in Hawai'i at some point but certainly not on the Big Island. I imagined myself on the sandy beach in Ka'anapali on Maui with gentle, warm breezes wafting over me while I lazily sipped MaiTais as the sun set into the ocean. I even purchased a condo in an ocean front resort on Maui. I spent my first night there as a grateful owner on December 31, 1998. I was so excited as I created my new life in paradise. Shortly after buying the condo I arranged with my employer to work from Maui so I began a six year commute back and forth between Maui and California. I was making my dream happen.

Then in 2005, a chain of events occurred which changed not only my direction, but my career and my entire life. To make a long story very short, I found myself out of a job, without a partner on a five acre property in the jungle of east Hawai'i. I came with only two suitcases of clothes. I guess someone forgot to tell me about the new plans because no one was more surprised than me to find myself here, wondering how the heck I got here.

Aloha, to learn what is not said...

In retrospect, my being here was probably the very best thing that could have happened to me considering

I wanted to shift the consciousness of the planet and I would probably be too distracted sitting on a Maui beach. In the days that followed, I learned so much about the land, the ocean, the jungle and the many creatures that shared space with me. I especially learned more about myself, my fears and my real reason for being on the planet. Thus I began my new life in paradise.

With Hawai'i being one of the most isolated land locations on the planet, there is a feeling that we are "in it together" that I have not felt before. As my ancestors knew, we are part of the earth, Gaia. Day by day as I lived on the island, I began to "learn" how we are all a part of a greater living system.

The five acre property I bought had some unusual characteristics which continuously revealed itself to me. The energy here was so intense that I typically would wake up each night around two o'clock in the morning with my entire body buzzing as if an electrical current was running through me. It was what the Hawaiians call, the Pele energy, the energy of the volcano and the energy was speaking to me through my body. I was shown how to live in the energy by allowing the current to run through me, give me what I needed to know and then lull me back to sleep. I had amazing dreams and when I was awake, I was guided to walk on the land barefooted. For a panty-hose wearing, high-heeled shoes businesswoman from Silicon Valley, this was no easy task. But I did it and I did it with reverence. The earth was telling me to walk on her skin with my skin.

During this time of knowing what was not said, I began a Native American practice of giving back to the land whenever I take from the land. So for all the food I purchased to eat from the farmers' market, I would gift the land with the seeds and skins from what I had eaten. Mind you, I was not planting the seeds or skins or vegetable tops, I was throwing the remains onto the land with gratitude for what I had received. Lo and hold, I had papayas, pineapples, lilikoi, avocados and tomatoes popping up all over. My black thumb is now green! My grandmother would be so proud.

I was also guided to create a water source on the land as this would be important. So I began to dig a hole in the lowest part of the property about thirty feet above sea level. Now, I did not literally begin to dig, I hired an excavator and operator to do it. It was challenging because we encountered "blue rock" which is the one of the hardest rocks on the planet. I began doubting my guidance, wondering if we would ever hit water and if we did, so what? Stressed as I was over the time and the cost, I continued forward with the Pele energy giving me strength. Finally after a few months' work, we encountered water. It was fresh and pure water; rain water filtered through the lava and running as an underground river through lava tubes to the ocean.

After a few days, we also found the water becoming brackish because the lava tubes would feed back ocean water through the same lava tubes at high tide. Thus an anchialine pond was born.

Anchialine ponds are naturally occurring ponds on the islands which are becoming polluted or dried up due to over development of the land. Well, I had a beautiful pond and within a year, I also had the rare Hawaiian Opae Ula (red shrimp) that are becoming endangered on the islands and they were thriving in the pond.

"Aloha, to see what cannot be seen…"

As Westerners came to the islands, the Hawaiian culture, language, spirituality and practices were outlawed and suppressed but were too lively to die out completely. They became *huna*, hidden, for hundreds of years, only practiced in remote jungle villages and mountain communities. As the Haole (those without breath, Ha) came, they sought to destroy what they did not understand. Much of Hawaiian history is distorted or disputed because it was not consistently passed on or it was changed so as not to attract attention. It is only recently that the Kahunas, the keepers of the knowledge, have dared to share their ancient wisdom. Slowly Hawaiian culture and spritually is recovering.

One of the old practices I was shown is the Hawaiian practice of Aloha which is sharing of the breath. "Alo" meaning sharing and "Ha" meaning breath. The Hawaiian greeting, *honi*, consists of placing the nostril gently beside that of the person greeted, a kind of sharing of breath, which is life. When an elder was passing, he would share his wisdom with his last breath, *Ha*. The breath that is life is also wisdom. The deeper spiritual meaning of *Ha* is soul or spirit.

Learning this, I became very conscious of my breath, how I was breathing and aware of the air I breathed, noting how rejuvenated I felt just breathing the fresh, clean air. Later I found out that the area I lived in had what was considered the freshest air on the planet. We are located on the eastern most tip of the island of Hawai'i. The closest land mass is Mexico. The trade winds blow from the east and as they travel the ocean, the air is purified with rain and sun until it reaches our shores. Isn't it wonderful that the wind and ocean collaborate to create pure air? Ancient Hawaiians called the trade winds *makani* or the life-giving spirit of air. No wonder just breathing this air is intoxicating, healthy and rejuvenating. In this clean air was spirit.

How beautiful to be part of an unseen system where sharing breath (our life sustaining essence) is a practice. Doesn't that make us very connected and interdependent? Doesn't that make us responsible for taking care of the air, land, ocean and neighbor?

To me this means helping to preserve the Hawaiian culture, legends, language, practices and spirituality. Similar to Native Americans, Hawaiians share their knowledge in a close circle. As Westerners, we have lots to learn about reverence of the land, air, water and life. Imagine if we could live in harmony with our environment, taking only what we need, giving back to replenish and caring for it as if our life depended on it!

Aloha, to know the unknowable...."

It is said that before she died, Queen Lili'uokalani found God. She passed her wisdom to her people through her definition of Aloha quoted above. My interpretation of her last phrase is that we can know the unknowable, God/Source/Supreme Being/Spirit, through It's every creation.

In July of 2007, a group of Lightworkers from all over the world were having a convention in the Kona area. One of the members lived close by and asked if she could invite a small group over to the land and possibly to swim in the pond. I said, "Yes, sure, it will be fun to have visitors." A couple of days later, about 17 people arrived. These Lightworkers are people who are Shamans, Healers, Energy Workers, Kahunas, Psychics and more. I was amazed at how "down to earth" they appeared. As we toured the land, they were making comments about the positive energy and what they were feeling.

We arrived at the top of the land rise above the pond, about forty feet above the water. This was the best vantage point to view the entire pond with the aqua blue to emerald green water and rocks. Suddenly the group started whispering and talking quietly to each other. I was in the dark about what was going on but I thought it was Lightworker stuff. After a couple of minutes, a woman began telling me what they were seeing. She asked, "Do you know what this pond is?" "I'm not sure," I said. She said, "It is a spiritual portal. There is lots of spiritual energy in the water. You are blessed." Whoa, spiritual energy in the pond? I knew that when anyone swam in the pond, they would have wonderful experiences, such as, feeling as if they were in the womb again, or feeling energized or rejuvenated.

Again to make a long story short, a Native American Shaman visiting me in 2008 and an Indonesian Guru in 2010 said similar things. The Shaman saw a strong medicine in the water and the Guru saw light orbs of spiritual energy in the water. Although I cannot see what they have seen, I believe it and I know I can feel it. Most people feel a sense of well-being, love and nurturing when swimming in the pond. It is unexplainable, yet real. My guidance to create this pond was certainly divinely inspired.

On this island which is much younger in geological terms than previously thought, I see the land forming as it must have formed millions of years ago. I see life coming into existence and then dying off rapidly with the lava flow. I see the pristine ocean and pure air blessing all the creatures that live here. I feel the energy of the earth flow through me.

And as Einstein has said, "I believe in Spinoza's God who reveals himself in the orderly harmony of what exists..." As I see the orderly harmony that exists in nature, I laugh at my worries about illness, death and dying. I am part of all that exists and as such, I am in tune to the natural cycle, not punished by it.

How can I know the unknowable if it is unknowable? Living on this island has taught me that intuitively I know my path without consciously knowing my path. How else would I have come here? It is having trust that I will learn what I need to know without being told, that I will be shown what I need to see without actually seeing it and to know what I must know without consciously knowing it. It takes surrender and trust and courage. Taking each day at a time, I learn to trust more and to surrender more.

Through this land called Hawai'i, I have learned what I did not know before, how to become in tune with the land and nature. I saw what I could not see before, the collaboration of nature to provide us with life-giving sustenance, as a compassionate mother who will nurture us if we allow her. We must give back and take care of her creation instead of only taking from her. And I came to know the "unknowable," the existence of God in everything and everyone. As I see the perfection around me created without effort, as I see the orderly harmony of nature, as I see new land being created, as I see water and air in pure form, I know the existence of God. Through this land, I know God and I know I am a part of God.

****

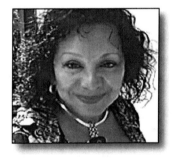

Sylvia Dolena is an entrepreneur, business consultant, executive coach and former leader at Hewlett-Packard, now living on the Big Island, Hawai'i. Throughout her career in high tech, Silicon Valley, her passion was to help people, especially women, develop as leaders and achieve their professional goals.

For over twenty-five years she has had many roles and responsibilities as business leader, operations manager, master consultant to large complex businesses world-wide; executive coach to senior global leaders and performance coach to business teams and work teams; global project manager; and leadership development educator. At Hewlett Packard she led several multi-million dollar businesses and managed strategic projects to improve business results and customer satisfaction. Sylvia has worked internationally with teams in Asia, Europe and the Americas.

As a Master Consultant and Executive Coach at HP, Sylvia coached over 40 executive leaders in the Winning Edge program and senior leaders in the "Leading Global Business Systems" programs. She also delivered over hundreds of Dynamic Leadership, Beyond Change, and Consultative Selling learning labs. Sylvia also coached an award-winning sales team.

While working at HP, Sylvia created Business Innovation Lab, as a consulting and coaching business in order to help small minority-owned businesses, startups and professionals be successful. Most recently, Sylvia partnered with a former HP co-worker, Pat Duran to create Accelerated Women Entrepreneurs to help women start their own businesses.

After moving to Hawai'i in 2005, Sylvia started Winning Edge University as a way of giving Hawai'i business people access to the education, experience and skills development typically available only to corporate executives. She has scaled many of the educational programs to fit the needs of Hawai'i business owners.

Sylvia also is developing a small organic farm in the Hawai'i jungle. This is the location she speaks of in her story. The farm will eventually be a natural, eco-retreat for people to have transformational experiences through facilitated visits, workshops or by working on the land. She is also partners in Hawaiian Cinema Productions, a film company, focused on producing documentaries for social and economic change in Hawai'i.

Sylvia's educational background includes two Executive MBAs: MS in Strategic Management of Technology Companies, joint project, Stanford University and IESE Business School in Barcelona; MBA, USC Marshall School of Business. She has an AS, BS, UC Sonoma in Computer Science. Sylvia's certifications include: Certified Professional and Executive Coach, Certified Master Business Consultant and Certified in Conversant Communications; trained in NLP and in NVC.

Sylvia's passion to help people is demonstrated in her community service:

- Developed and delivered training, coaching and mentorship for Latino students at risk through the Digital Bridge Educational project in California

- Delivered leadership and communication workshops to minority youths locally

- Established GraceNet Silicon Valley Chapter as an educational and networking forum for professional business women who are in transition due to business downturn, downsizing or other economic disruptions

- Coach to Director of a non-profit school for minority students preparing for college

- Coach to women who are in transition and looking for a life and/or career change

Contact: sylviadolena@yahoo.com 808 965-1899

Websites: www.winningedgeuniv.com   www.pelelani.com
www.hawaiiancinema.com

Hawai'i has the key and that key is ALOHA.

The meaning of Aloha comes from the heart and is given freely.

The spiritual meaning to each letter of the word aloha:

A stands for AKAHAI, meaning kindness, expressed with tenderness.

L is for LOKAHI, meaning unity, expressed with harmony.

O is for OLU'OLU, meaning agreeable, expressed with pleasantness.

H stands for HA'AHA'A, meaning humility, expressed with modesty.

A stands for AHONUI, meaning patient and persevering.

Written by Hawaiian poet and philosopher Pilahi Paki, a renowned and beloved linguist. Adopted by the Hawai'i Legislature in 1986 ([§5-7.5] Aloha Spirit)

Examples of Aloha in My Life

Dalani Tanahy

I was once taught by a kumu hula, that the word 'Aloha' was so sacred it was never used casually. A more proper greeting would be '`Ano `ai'. At The Cultural Learning Center at Ka`ala where I work, our kupuna taught us more about that sacred aspect. He said that interpreted, 'alo' means the face or, to face directionally, such as the face of the kalo leaf as its looks towards the sun. It also means to be present, in the presence of something. 'Ha' meaning the breath of life, inferring that creator who gave us all life. Thus Aloha would mean, 'in the presence of god'.

When we were taught the proper way to greet each other, not with a kiss, but with a 'honi', again, it inferred this breath of life. With foreheads touching, each person would, through their noses, not mouths, inhale and then 'haaaaaaa' and exchange the pure breath of life, bonding them together as friends and ohana. Taking the thought even further, the bamboo flutes and gourd whistles played by the Hawaiians were all played through the breath of the nose, thus ensuring the purest cleanest sounds.

I know that Aloha is not to be found only on our fair shores, but have seen it on the other side of the world as well. I travelled to Egypt a number of times, and after spending that time there, could only come away with one description of the people...'Wow, they have plenty aloha!' So what was that 'Aloha Factor'? What was the commonality? A particular openness, a generosity unfeigned; a welcoming smile and a naturally hospitable nature. When I visited American Samoa, I experienced the same thing. People who took immense joy in making sure you ate more than any normal human could. People who, when you tried to give them thank you gifts for hosting you, gave you more gifts just because you came! Again, I could only say 'wow, they have plenty aloha'.

Back home in the Islands, I must admit, I have seen a dilution of the aloha. I have seen children growing up without being encouraged in their natural tendencies to share and to love without prejudice. I see the lack of love and aloha in families and homes, and replaced with self centeredness, avarice and attachments to things and ideals that have little or no value.

So what is aloha to me? What were the examples that I saw as a child and that influenced my life? I would have to say my Grandmothers. I was fortunate to have both my paternal and maternal grandparents around, well into my young adult years, losing my last surviving grandpa when I was in my mid forties. My all-the- time grandma was my dad's mom, Julia Prager, who lived near us in San Diego. In her small humble home with the giant yard. I ate fresh baked whole wheat bread and fruity jello salads and dark rich beans and sausage. We ate loquats from her tree and fed her fat gold fish in their ponds. For my birthdays she would bake my favorite chocolate potato cake with homemade frosting sprinkled with walnuts. When I flew to Hawaii to visit my maternal Grandma, Emily Enos, Grandma Prager would fill a coffee tin with my favorite peanut cookies to eat on the trip. When I arrived in La`ie, Grandma and Grandpa Arthur Enos would take us to lunch at the Church College of Hawaii, where they supervised the cafeteria. They would have the cook make us some hamburgers as a treat before we went home to have the real feast. Grandma was also teaching the international cooking class at the school, so we could be sure to taste some rare exotic thing we had never tried before. Grandpa had a pink stripped jeep with a fringe on top and we loved nothing more than driving around the neighborhood with him, smiling and waving to everyone.

I discovered that food and feeding people is so intrinsic to aloha through the examples of my grandmothers. What other examples did I see? Both of them exemplified humility and service to others. They were both very active in church, doing genealogy and serving in whatever capacities they were asked to. They checked on people, took food to people, called people to say hello and cheer them up. They loved all us grandkids equally and without reservation, and took it upon themselves to gently chasten us when it seemed like we needed it. Grandma Enos was very artistic and taught me to sew and paint. Grandma Prager was a wonderful horticulturist and gave me a great appreciation for learning about plants and tending to them. Both grandmas were very spiritual and taught me the importance of staying true to my convictions, whether or not others agreed, but to be humble and a peacemaker as well.

Looking back, I really miss my grandmas, and grandpas, and wish that I had spent more time letting them know how much I appreciated the lessons they taught us grandkids. I will never forget Grandma Enos' sly lessons on modesty, when she would call out "how deep is my valley?" if our shirts were a little too low... before we even had any valley to speak of! I will never forget Grandma Prager out in the back of her wild but organized garden, taking a big bite of a Natal plum, which I had always assumed was deathly poisonous because of its milky sap, and despite our horror of impending doom for grandma, saying to us with a straight face, "no it won't kill you if you eat it."

Looking forward, as a grandma myself now, with two grandchildren here, one in heaven and more on the way I'm sure, I wonder if I will exemplify even a fraction of the aloha I saw in my grandmas. I may have to hone those skills a little more. I know there are things that do not come naturally to me, but I know I have some qualities that I think, with a little work, I might rise to the knee-caps of my larger-than-life grandmas and their unforgettable examples of living aloha.

****

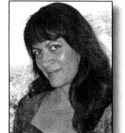

Dalani Tanahy is a native of San Diego California with maternal roots from Waikapu, Maui and is a direct descendant of Edward Bailey and Emily Kane of Wailuku. Growing up, she spent enough summers in La`ie with her grandparents, Emily and Arthur Enos, that she knew she would return to the 'homeland' one day.

Currently living in Makaha with her 'tribe', she is an avid surfer and body boarder, a practitioner of the art of Hawaiian

Kapa making and works for the non-profit organization, Ka`ala Farm Inc, in Wai`anae. As a writer, she was once a reporter and profiler for H20 magazine, where she usually wrote about women in the waves and interviewed famous surfers like the Queen of Makaha, Rell Sunn. In her free time… okay, she has no free time, but hopes to someday, and would like to visit India to see the Taj Mahal and South Africa to see the jumping Great White Sharks.

Success Comes From Aloha

Holan Nakata

Starting a business can be difficult in itself. With no formal business education, setting up an operation at the age of 19 can seem almost next to impossible.

By the grace of God, my business thrives and I'm in my fourth year. It is no coincidence that I started my first business in Hawai'i. The Aloha that people shared helped me on my journey.

I was studying at a university in Northern California. I stayed in California during the breaks and I called my family from time to time. Eventually, I was informed that my family was facing financial setbacks. My father told me not to worry but I flew back to Hawai'i to support my family anyway.

The dynamics of my family are no better or worse than other families. It was just different.

My mother died when I was young and my father was left with two young boys to raise. My father did not remarry. A mother is a special role that three guys cannot fulfill but we did what we could to do our part to make the family work. No matter how much time passes, there is a little pain in each and every one of us. A little help from each of us goes a long ways.

I experienced my first taste of a few financial setbacks. Money was owed, bills weren't being paid, and the amount that was spent on food was less than two hundred dollars a month, and that was for a family of three. We survived off selling possessions and the social security checks given by the government until my brother reached adulthood.

At times like that, sometimes all you can do is pray. Without a college education, a job would not be enough to support my family. We kept our situation private but people that have been through it can sense it. Family would drop off food and friends would invite us over for lunch or dinner. Some just stopped by to talk. Their actions, their Aloha gave us the strength to move forward and look for a better tomorrow.

We knew we could not rely on sellingpossessions. With the money we saved up, I converted a storage space into an office, registered a company, and created a website where I shared my story.

In my first week of business I made ten dollars. I was overjoyed. In six months, I made enough to cover both the business and living expenses. Customers shared their words of encouragement. Some were entrepreneurs that shared their own business experiences. Others shared getting through difficult times. Many mentioned how my story on my website touched their hearts. It was a reminder that we all go through tough times but it is the Aloha we share that helps everyone move forward.

I loved every part of business in Hawai'i. Depositing money to the bank was more than dropping off money. It was a time to smile and share about life. That was aloha.

People that I once perceived as competitors visited me and I learned to set aside my differences and be friendly. Somebody told me, Hawai'i is such a small place, and there's enough business to go around, and as America was facing a financial crisis, we found strength in moral support with others in the same industry. I wondered if this type of Aloha is unique to Hawai'i. Overall, I thank God that this where I started my first business, the Aloha helped me get through the challenges all entrepreneurs face.

We can run into people we don't know. The concept of Aloha tells us that they're not strangers. We can talk about faith, politics, and culture and even if we have our differences, we find common ground in Aloha.

Is it the beauty of the islands with radiant weather that brings out the Aloha in people? Is Aloha from the culture that the native Hawaiians preserved? Did Aloha originate from the melting pot of people of different cultures that settled to call Hawai'i their home? Maybe the concept of Aloha starts with a small group of people and it catches on to the world around them around like contagious laughter. Either way, Hawai'i and Aloha holds a special place in my heart that I take with me where ever I go.

****

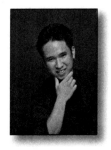

I ulu no ka lala i ke kumu

The reach of a tree's branches depends on its trunk.
A family's unconditional love strengthens
each one to succeed.

Sharing is Aloha

Gloria Cohen

The word "aloha" has many meanings in the Hawaiian language. Most common would be *hello, goodbye* and *love*. Aloha, however, is also a way of life. It's about family, giving and sharing. The goal is to have the Aloha Spirit.

When asked by Anolia to contribute to this project, I had to stop and think about how to approach what aloha means to me. Even though this word is in my everyday language, it became immediately clear while having a difficult time deciding what to write, that I am living aloha and therefore the task became describing my aloha life.

I have been traveling to the Hawaiian Islands for over 25 years, very unusual for someone from the East Coast. My first visits were to O`ahu, and I still have memories of my first trips: the scent of Plumeria in the air, of flowers that had showered from the trees to the ground; memories of the color changes in the ocean and in the sky, the air itself had a way of embracing me. It was my sense that this place, Hawai`i, was sharing aloha.

I spent several years traveling to O`ahu, sometimes working in the fashion or beauty industry and often on vacation. I spent a lot of time on the North Shore where the amazing surf is, in total awe. After that I ventured to Maui and loved the lagoons where the dolphins would come to play. I have long felt that it was important to my wellbeing to spend time in the Hawaiian Islands; for me they have a peaceful, healing quality.

When I was in my early working years, I spent a lot of time in the Caribbean and California on photo shoots. But the *only* place I spent my own hard-earned dollars for vacation was Hawai`i. Now I spend most of my time on the Garden Island of Kaua`i, overlooking the sea where I watch whales migrate and dolphins swim in great numbers. This is aloha all around me, a gift from Mother Nature.

I have had many successful careers in my life, and I realize now that sharing all the knowledge I have acquired from each section of my life is aloha. I was always willing to share what I knew or what I had learned, I am good at this. I was never afraid or worried that someone would try to get my job with the information I was sharing. I'm a great believer that "what goes around comes around." Sharing is aloha; these islands have given to me, and now I am giving back.

I have been an artist my whole life in one form or another, from painting, oils and water color—to being a fashion makeup artist working on the covers and editorial pages of top fashion magazines with photographers like Irving Penn, Richard Avedon and many others, to being an award-winning fine jewelry designer. I am also the author of *The Pregnant Woman's Beauty Book* published by William Morrow many years ago plus many other projects from that time period. In more recent times, with my husband, I have owned part of a restaurant in New York City, a 200 room hotel on the ocean in Hawai`i, and a wholesale flower distribution center in Southern California. I feel it is important to share with others that change is good and one should not be afraid to try the next thing. Learning to trust that you can do it and be good at it is trusting the aloha within you, trusting that you can achieve your goals.

Today, besides creating my art and jewelry, I am the publisher of the only award-winning 100% food magazine in the state of Hawai`i: *Edible Hawaiian Islands*. This magazine is unusual in that it is a statewide publication, almost all other magazines in Hawai`i are island centric, more about this magazine later. As an artist, I am involved in every possible way on every page, to make sure the aloha, the knowledge and the beauty of where I live comes through.

In 2001, I had an unusual experience, which caused me to stop and think very seriously about the world and my part in it. I knew I had to do something, I was meant to do something. I just didn't know what. It took a number of years, and then it happened: I discovered the Edible Community magazines, and, literally, a light bulb went off in my head. This is a community of publishers who own their own territory but stay together under one umbrella; this gives us all a national presence as well as a support team. When I signed on five years ago I was publication number 29. Today there are almost 70 Edible publications across the United States and Canada.

Immediately, I started thinking, "The Hawaiian Islands are all about agriculture, how perfect. I could help educate people on the importance of eating and supporting local. It is my turn to share and give aloha to as many people as I could reach." My dream is to connect the dots between our islands, telling the stories of what each island has to offer, each one being so different from the next and having unique resources. After 9/11, I realized that here in the middle of the Pacific Ocean, we all need to know what is available nearby.

When one hears the words "the Hawaiian Islands," images of beauty come to mind. We see paradise in the middle of the Pacific, deep blue seas, lush mountains and rain forests, clean fresh air, luscious exotic fruits, fish with names you can't pronounce. In the past these islands were all about eating local. We need to encourage this again, to take pride and pleasure in local, seasonal, authentic foods and the many culinary traditions of the Hawaiian Islands.

When the first issue of my magazine came out, we took the magazines to our local outdoor farmers' market and started handing them out to the small local farmers. Some of these farmers had tears in their eyes. One woman said to me, "No one has ever paid attention to us before. *Mahalo.*" This brought tears to my eyes.

Aloha for me is being able to celebrate the family farmers, bakers, fisherman, ranchers, poultry farmers, local chefs and the rest of the community for their dedication to producing the highest quality fresh and seasonal foods. My "Aloha Mission" is to highlight these people and their efforts towards a more sustainable and safe food system in all of the Hawaiian Islands. This is why I produce and publish *Edible Hawaiian Islands*.

****

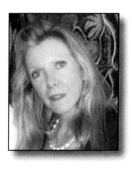

Gloria Cohen is Publisher/Editor-in-Chief of *Edible Hawaiian Islands Magazine*

More aloha at
www.edibleHawaiianislands.com

Aloha from a Health Perspective

Cheryl Toyofuku

"Your pre-malignant colon is going to be the primary cause of your future health challenges." My Honolulu physician with his kind, yet penetrating eyes spoke these words gently to me. How can this be? I was only in my mid-thirties, felt okay and as an oncology certified registered nurse, I thought I was doing what I needed to do to stay healthy. I did remember that an aunt, uncle and several cousins on the paternal side of my family were diagnosed with colon cancer at young ages. A small thought began to formulate in my mind that perhaps this was something that I needed to take seriously. My hectic, stressful, fast-food lifestyle was probably a contributor to this health consequence.

A few days later, in the outpatient oncology unit that I worked in, I was sitting with a patient's family member. He came in to donate some blood platelets for his relative who was diagnosed with leukemia. Our unit was often bustling with activity as part of a major medical institution in Hawai'i. In the small, cold room that we conversed in, I was monitoring his blood that was being removed from one of his arms then going through a blood cell separator machine that separated his blood cells, so that only his blood platelets could be retrieved into a small pouch. The rest of his blood would then be returned to him in his other arm.

During our conversation, I noticed that the small bag was being filled with platelets and plasma that appeared quite viscous, cloudy and sticky. Usually the liquid collected in the pouch is a clear light yellow. Out of curiosity, I inquired with him what he had for breakfast. He replied that it was a special Hawaiian loco-moco with eggs, portugese sausage, gravied hamburger patty on top of white rice, along with a chocolate shake. I realized then that what I was seeing was all the fat that was oozing out of his blood along with the platelets into the bag. I also wondered what my blood looked like.

The elderly medical doctor that had given me the new-found revelation about my colon was known to be associated with western and eastern medicine. Interestingly, he was also a complementary health practitioner who utilized innovative diagnostic technology and treatment options from all over the world. I eventually began to work with him part-time and along with my own quest for health answers, it became a passion to learn what it takes to truly have a sense of health, vitality and wellness. On this health journey, I've learned a lot through association with other health advocates, organizations, health resources and companies, native and ministry healers. I have been impacted the most with my research into what my Creator says about this.

A most intimate moment occurred at the beginning of mankind. It was when the Creator of heaven and earth breathed into man's nostrils the breath of life (Genesis 2:7). Man became a living being with this face to face encounter with God.

In Hawai'i, the special greeting of "Aloha" suggests an intimate exchange of love and respect, whether it is with one other person or to a group. "Alo" ("face to face" or "in the presence") and "ha" ("life" or "breath") is a reminder to me of the wonder of how we were created. Among the different meanings of the word "Aloha," this back-to-creation perspective evokes in me a deep respect for God as the Creator of human existence and for each other as His creation. It has become an attitude or a way of life for myself and others. In Hawai'i, this lifestyle of gratitude, honor and respect is sometimes called "The Aloha Spirit".

It is with this grateful mindset, that I am fully embracing my home state's destiny and purpose. A transforming work is being birthed here in these beautiful islands. In the midst of tremendous challenges, there is a small group of proactive revolutionists rising up to fulfill the calling that is unfolding through revelation from the Creator. Faithful believers are uniting as a true ohana or family who love God, each other and the aina, the land of Hawai'i. This family is emerging from all walks of life with each individual member of this ohana contributing his or her unique gifting to complete the tapestry of Hawai'i's destiny.

As part of this growing community, I am recognizing my role as a mother, grandmother, daughter, sister, friend, RN and health advocate. My passion and desire has been to help myself and my ohana while on our journey towards optimal health and healing in spirit, soul and body. I have learned that dependence on the Creator as the Master Teacher, Great Physician and Compassionate Healer is the key to transforming lives from sickness to health. I am reminded that Jesus is the Bread of Life, the Living Water and the Light of the World. He is the Healer, Deliverer and Savior. He still heals miraculously today with healing signs and wonders following those who believe.

Respect for God as my Creator has taught me to have a respect for my body for it is fearfully and wonderfully made (Psalm 139:13-14). I am reminded that God, in designing man, created me with a spirit, soul and body (1Thessalonians 5:23). As His creation, He desires me to be completely yielded up to His will. His Holy Spirit in union with my spirit will govern my soul and then use my body as a means of expressing His purposes. His everlasting love for me is expressed through His desire for me to be abundantly healthy in all areas. This has become my everyday Aloha as I recognize my exciting destiny as a fifty five year old grandmother, to share God's love and Aloha to others. In order to do this, health care reform and transformation begins with me first, not with the government, medical system or others.

Therefore, I am learning to hear His voice and to listen to His prescription for me to remove toxins in my spirit, soul and body. He encourages me to nourish my spirit and mind with His wondrous Word and to feed my physical body with His bountiful healthy nutrients that He supplies on this earth. He renews me with His Holy Spirit and transforms me with His truths and promises. He continually reminds me with the revelation that health and healing in my own life is my kuleana or responsibility. This progressive transformation and reformation in my spirit, soul and body will only manifest with the revelation of Who created me, why He created me and how He created me. This marvelous revelation has changed my perception on what I am responsibly required to do in order to be healthy in my spirit, soul and body.

Every new health revelation produces a greater sense of awe at this One God, who allows it to be revealed. New health and healing discoveries are being uncovered even now with ways to remove toxins (spiritually, mentally, emotionally and physically), restore hydration (to quench our thirst in our spirit, soul and body) and renew our spirit, mind and body. Our immune system in all areas becomes stronger and overall longevity is increased. Our heavenly Father's instructions, grace, hope, faithfulness and everlasting love empowers us to believe and have faith to live in His anointing, healing and glory.

Beloved, I pray that you may prosper in all things and be in health, just as your soul prospers.

3 John 1:2

I wish you true health and wellness, the Aloha way according to God's design for you and me. On this journey, you and I are being encouraged to develop the wise healthy choices, habits and commitment that will honor ourselves and our Creator. Together we can surf the Hawaiian wave of wellness that has approached the shores of our beautiful islands of Aloha!

****

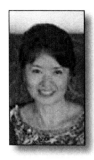 **Cheryl Toyofuku** is a registered nurse (R.N.) graduated with a Bachelors of Science in Nursing from the University of Hawai'i. As a Registered Nurse, former Oncology Certified Nurse and former Associate Director for the Foundation for East-West Medicine, she has transitioned to assisting family and friends with more nutritional, natural and non-toxic programs of health care. She is the founder of *Health Journey Hawai'i*, to assist herself and others while on the journey towards optimal health and healing in spirit, soul and body. HJH was established for the purpose of providing health options, perspectives and general health and healing principles.

For more information or to contact her, visit her website: www.healthjourneyHawaii.rr.com

He kēhau hoʻomaʻemaʻe ka aloha

Love is like a cleansing dew.
The cleansing power of Aloha can soothe and heal.
Love removes hurt. Love conquers all.

Aloha the Mirror of God's Love

Lee Miller Lane

Hawai'i has always been a sought after destination. I grew up in Pittsburgh, Pennsylvania in a dysfunctional family like many people. Consequently, I spent my youth dreaming of warm and exotic places like Hawai'i. I imagined if I were somewhere else I would be happier than I was as a child. After college I was hired by an airline and visited Hawai'i as often as possible for vacation. I found Hawai'i magical. My first impression was the sweet intoxicating smell of the lei's when you step off the plane. The warm balmy breezes and happy friendly people made me feel welcome and filled with me with joy! That was my first impression and memories of the Aloha State.

In 2003 my husband, Kelly, got a job offer in Honolulu. I loved Hawai'i; however, I was afraid to leave California and move so far across a big ocean away from friends and family. I knew with children and the cost of living we would be unable to visit the mainland very often.

We had only been to the island twice in almost eight years. What I did not know, was that moving to Hawai'i and catching the spirit of Aloha would change our lives 365 degrees! Moving was absolutely the best decision we have ever made.

When came in July 2003 we had two small boys under 4 years old and one on the way.

I was seven months pregnant. We were coming here for a new start. We were not married yet and our lives were tumultuous at best. As dysfunctional as my childhood was my adult life was worse. Kelly and I both were so emotionally wounded as children we were incapable of being good parents or partners to each other.

I truly believe God himself planned and arranged our move to Hawai'i to bring healing and solace to our lives. Hawai'i was our last chance. The meaning of Aloha has become much deeper and more profound as we have experienced real and eternal change in our lives as the Spirit revealed Himself to us.

Within a few weeks of arriving I was hired by a local Christian radio station despite being very pregnant at the time. The station manager kept scratching his head and saying "I don't know why I am hiring you, you will probably not return after the baby is born." This was evidence to me that this was one of our first miracles! It was there at the radio station that God opened my eyes to His spirit and the true meaning of Aloha. I met many people - but I was most attracted to the people that I met that had this aura about them of gentleness and kindness. They were calm and gracious no matter what was going on at the station or in their lives.

I soon discovered there was a profound difference between people who know the Lord and have a relationship with Jesus than those that do not. The difference became evident and very clear to me. The former live Aloha! They attract people to them because of the light that they carry inside of them. It shines out to the world through their eyes and actions.

I wanted that light and set out on a journey to acquire it for myself and my floundering family. I was on a mission and what happened next was yet another miracle! Kelly began to want the change I wanted so desperately too! He followed me in our pursuit of the kingdom of God. We started going to Church. We opened our house for Bible studies and God provided mentors and teachers that actually came to us to share God's Word and the spirit of Aloha. After being discipled for awhile Kelly had the opportunity and privilege to water baptize his own family. What an awesome experience!

Right from inception of moving to Hawai'i, God's Spirit started working on us and we started to see small miracles and change for the better in our lives. Aloha is a word in the Hawaiian language that has numerous meanings both as a single word and when used in context with other words. Aloha is commonly used to mean love. It is used to express compassion, regret or sympathy. Deeper meaning and sacredness comes from experiencing Aloha which we found out for ourselves.

"On a spiritual level, aloha is an invocation of the Divine that dwells within and without." Aloha [Alo = presence, front, face] + [hā = breath] = The presence of (Divine) Breath.'"

As the Spirit began revealing and healing our relationship, we both became hungry to understand the Spirit even more! It became an unquenchable thirst for the things of God. I started Bible school four years ago and have completed my Bachelors in Theology. I am currently working on my Masters. The spirit of Aloha, God's divine breath, literally has saved our relationship, marriage and life! Our children are firmly planted in God's Word and we have peace of mind that these Children will serve God the rest of their lives. They will inherit the Kingdom of God and live forever in Paradise.

Kelly and I got married at the Lagoons in Kapolei a year after we moved to the islands. My husband had been married twice before and thoroughly believed at the time the institution of marriage itself is why both relationships failed. However, God had other plans. When we accepted Christ, we decided to be all in and do life His way! We stopped living in sin, got married and surrendered our lives to the Lord. Our relationship has been transformed by that simple act of obedience. I actually love and respect my husband more, today than when I met him or even married him almost seven years ago.

We have a strong happy marriage today and we are a living breathing testimony of the transforming healing power of God's love and Aloha. The words God and Aloha are a mirrored image for us. People fall in love with Hawai'i because they experience the essence of God which is love and which also means Aloha. This is one of the most special places on earth! We have made Hawai'i our permanent home here on earth because of blessings and transformation we have received from living Aloha.

We believe so much in the transformational healing power of Aloha that we started an evangelical ministry together. We want to share the healing we have experienced from floundering to flourishing, literally from hell to well.

The spirit and essence of Aloha is life changing. I received the vision from the Holy Spirit in November 2008 to begin the ministry. He Reigns is all about putting God first in all areas of our lives! Letting the spirit transform and heal through "Aloha - The presence of (Divine) Breath," is our message and vision for He Reigns.

Our website was created to be a communication tool similar to social network sites with a cause to be *"The Site to Unite Gods People."* Hosea 4:6 *"My people perish for lack of knowledge"* is one of my favorite scriptures probably because before moving to Hawai'i we had no knowledge of God's love or healing power. We had to move here to experience it.

We believe by using technology and the internet we can share God's healing power and the meaning of Aloha with the world. People do not necessarily have to visit or move to Hawai'i to catch the divine breath that is revealed in the essence of Aloha – they can experience it through people unified in His spirit – sharing his love with one another from wherever they are in the world.

The most important transformation people can manifest in their lives is becoming a living testimony, sharing their light and love freely. So, when we share Gods love and plan for salvation with others we are actually sharing a future and hope for their soul in paradise. We are sharing the message and essence of Aloha!

Our ministries primary purpose is to advance the Kingdom of God by winning souls for Heaven. We want people to know they do not have to stay stuck and hopeless. They do not have to be another unhappy statistic. The World does not teach righteousness. God gave us the Bible – which stands for Basic Instruction Before Leaving Earth. Living righteously means knowing God's Word and being obedient to what pleases the Lord. Trusting and obeying God pleases Him, which then creates a happier more abundant life. We know first hand we are living breathing miracles. We want people to understand they can be miracles too. Our choices ultimately decide what we experience on earth and it decides where we will spend eternity.

"But seek first His kingdom and His righteousness, and all these things will be added to you." When we put God first in our lives EVERYTHING changes.
- Matthew 6:33

Jesus looked at them and said, *"With man this is impossible, but with God all things are possible."*
- Matthew 19:26

What was impossible for us, fixing our marriage and our hearts was easy for God. We just had to give Him the reigns of our lives. When He Reigns – We Reign!

United speaking with one heart, mind and spirit, the message of Aloha can transform the world and grow the Kingdom of God here on earth and in Heaven. He Reigns is where faith, fun and fellowship meet. Together we can do BIG things for God that truly make a difference! "He Reigns, We Serve and You Matter," is our motto. We invite you to join us and spread God's message of Aloha around the Globe!

****

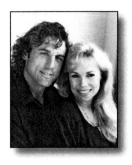

Lee Miller Lane

Founder & Visionary

He Reigns Christian Network

www.HeReignsHawaii.com

www.HeReignsGlobal.com

Aloha Brings Us All Together

Leslie Tyson

It always amuses me when it comes to ordering something from abroad. Inevitably, the operator will always quote a higher shipping rate than for any of the 48 contiguous states, stating that Hawai'i falls in the international category. Assuredly, the higher prices can be accredited to our location, smack dab in the middle of the Pacific Ocean, but that is just one aspect that sets Hawai'i apart from the other states.

Hawai'i is a melting pot of ethnicities and cultures, which gives our state a unique flavor. Its people have come from many countries, all with a dream for a better life. We, as a people, have come together, blending cultures, customs and even language. Someone visiting from the mainland (continental U.S.) will quickly notice that the islanders have a distinct dialect—something we call Pidgin English. Originally, it was a way of communicating that used simplified speech and even integrated words from the mother tongue of the various residents who came from Portugal, Japan, China, Philippines, Korea and many other countries. Today, it has become part of our culture.

My great-grandfather first arrived here over 120 years ago—before Hawai'i even became a state. As with most immigrants at that time, he came seeking an opportunity to make a fortune, with the hopes of returning to Japan to make life better with his newfound prosperity. However, life was difficult and the labor was hard. Like most, he was never able to return to Japan, and so was destined to remain in Hawai'i to raise his family. Many of the immigrants had come to work as a laborer in the cane fields. Hence a song titled *Hole Hole Bushi* (pronounced hō-lĕ hō-lĕ büshi) was composed by my former Japanese song teacher, Harry Minoru Urata. "Bushi" is the Japanese word for melody or song, and "hole hole" is the Hawaiian word for the dried sugarcane leaves that were manually stripped from the stalks. It was a song the workers would sing out in the fields, bemoaning the backbreaking work and measly compensation.

As a fourth-generation Japanese American, I have seen how this hardship has over the years served to unite the people of Hawai'i. I have been blessed to see the fruits of my ancestors' labor. Through their perseverance and determination, they have created a life here in Hawai'i for all the family to enjoy. There is a commonality that has brought us all together over the years — one that allows us to share our customs, blending our traditions to form the unique culture of Aloha.

****

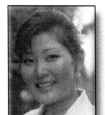

Leslie Tyson, owner and founder of Smart Solutions 24-7, Leslie M. Tyson happily provides customized services through Virtual Assistance support for her clients. With a penchant for business, she continues to seek new opportunities to expand, as a means to support various non-profit organizations in her community.

She endeavors to use her position in the market place as an outreach to connect other entrepreneurs with the same vision to impact their community in a powerful way, bringing hope to all.

She credits her Lord and Creator for the wonderful opportunities that abound as a work-at-home wife to husband Morris, and daughter Chelsea. Her life mission is to make a difference in the lives of others, while she still has breath. Not wanting to waste any time, she strives to make the most of every moment—balancing work, fun times with family, homeschool activities, and personal pursuits, such as learning to speak Russian and seeing how many more years she can complete the Honolulu Marathon.

Ho'omoe wai kāhi ke kāo'o

Let us all travel together like water flowing in one direction
Live in harmony with other people
and the world around you.

Aloha through the True Spirit of Bayanihan

Charlie Y. Sonido, M.D.

"Aloha" and "Bayanihan" are two distinct words emanating from two different languages and cultures yet both embody the essence of goodwill, compassion and service. Hence it would not be inaccurate to say that rendering a service in the spirit of Bayanihan, a Filipino word from the Islands of the Philippines which means "to work together" or "to help carry each other's load," is analogous to one performed in the spirit of Aloha. The Bayanihan Clinic Without Walls (BCWW) is a charitable organization composed of volunteer doctors, dentists, nurses, pharmacists and other allied health care professionals who banded together to answer a need in the community – free medical service to the uninsured and underprivileged members of the community. For us volunteers, this is the way we live in the spirit of Aloha or Bayanihan.

A Free Clinic

The Bayanihan Clinic Without Walls (BCWW) is a non-profit community based health care project established in 1997. Its mission is to provide free primary health care services to those in the community who have no health coverage and are currently classified as indigent and/or underprivileged, including the homeless, newly-arrived immigrants and migrants especially from the Pacific Islands.

BCWW was bestowed 501(c) (3) privileges as a non-profit organization in April 1999. The term *bayanihan* refers to a distinctive Filipino spirit of communal cooperation or effort to achieve a particular goal or to solve a common problem.

Common Background

Tracing the history of BCWW to its inception invariably leads to the Philippine Medical Association of Hawai'i (PMAH). Most, if not all, of BCWW's volunteer physicians are also members of PMAH. Many came to the U.S. from the Philippines during the 1970s and as newly-arrived immigrants, they struggled with the rigors of medical training, raising families as well as adjusting to a new culture in their host county and a new way of life. It was during these trying times, especially during medical residency training and, after that, starting their own practices, that strong bonds were formed.

Violeta Soriano, PMAH Historian and Auxiliary President noted in the PMAH's 30th Anniversary souvenir publication, "They strongly felt the need for an association of Filipino doctors not only for the friendship of their colleagues but for mutual support as well as the sharing and advancement of medical expertise and knowledge. It was an idea whose time has come and only needed someone like Dr. Etty Bautista, a physiatrist with the Tripler Army Medical Center, to lead the efforts and make the dream a reality. Hence at its first meeting at Tripler Hospital's Orchid Room, on August 30, 1978, PMAH was born."

Out of the shared obstacles and challenges, these doctors bonded together in the true spirit of *bayanihan*, drawing strength from each other and sharing their resources as a team. "We had to band together to survive the hardships of training, the language barrier, and adjusting to life in the U.S. like one big family", says Dr. Herita Yulo, BCWW co-founder and its first president.

Meeting The Need

In August 22, 1996 a federal law was passed that denied medical benefits to some 800-1000 immigrants who were then enrolled under the QUEST medical insurance program. In response, the Hawai'i State Legislature appropriated monies to provide benefits and medical services for those who no longer qualified for Medicaid. The monies were meant to compensate community health centers for providing health care to medically uninsured immigrants and others who were ineligible for Medicaid or the State Quest medical insurance program.

Due to the impact of the 1996 federal law upon the community, an appeal was made to the medical community, imploring the aid of physicians in private practice to volunteer their services. More than thirty physicians of Filipino ancestry answered the call for help. In April 17, 1997, the PMAH, under the leadership of Dr. Charlie Sonido, initiated the Bayanihan Clinic Without Walls project. "I suggested that we use the words "without walls" to reflect the fact that the organization had no actual headquarters, office or physical structure from where it operated and from where services were dispensed to those in need. The services were delivered out of individual private offices and clinics of the volunteer physicians," says BCWW co-founder Dr. Sonido. By October 1997, free dental services were added to its basic health services. In 1998, the list of volunteers increased to forty nine representing thirteen subspecialties. The current list of subspecialties have expanded and include Family Medicine, Internal Medicine, Pediatrics, Obstetrics/Gynecology, Cardiology, Gastroenterology, Nephrology, Ear, Nose & Throat (ENT), Anesthesiology, General Surgery,

Orthopedic Surgery, Plastic Surgery, Cardiothoracic Surgery, Ophthalmology, Urology, Neurology, Oncology, Pulmonary Medicine, Dermatology, Geriatrics, Infectious Disease, Psychiatry, Psychology, Radiology and Dentistry.

Free services are provided for those who meet the following eligibility requirements: 1. Immigrants who entered the U.S. on or after August 22, 1996 and who meet Medicaid or QUEST income and asset eligibility criteria. 2. Legal immigrants without medical insurance who have been in the U.S. for not more than one year. 3. Migrants from the Compact of Free Association (COFA) – Federated States of Micronesia, Republic of Marshall Islands, Republic of Palau - who meet Medicaid and QUEST income and asset eligibility but are rejected for coverage by these programs. 4. Those classified as financially indigent based on the Federal Poverty Level Guidelines.

"Although the qualification requirements haven't changed much through the years, we have recently set up an adhoc committee to review these criteria and to update them, if necessary," says current BCWW President Dr. Nicanor Joaquin.

Annually, BCWW participates actively in free community health fairs in Lanai, Molokai, Maui, Kauai, Oahu, and the Big Island. Needy residents receive free health screenings, physical exams, dental examinations and health education. For years BCWW has been a regular participant in the Filipino Festival held annually at the Kapiolani Park in Honolulu providing free hypertension and diabetes screening and counseling, eye examinations, bone density measurements, limited physical and massage therapy, mental health counseling as well as distributing health education kits and other giveaways. BCWW members have also participated in many international medical missions and touched the lives of thousands more. In 2008, the organization initiated a Health Education Promotion project to enhance public awareness of the importance of good health by publishing in local newspapers original materials and articles written by BCWW members on some common illnesses such as gout, hypertension, and sexually transmitted diseases. To date, it has provided free health screening tests and medical services to some 6000 indigent patients.

"Leading these dedicated physician-volunteers has truly been an honor", says BCWW immediate past president Dr. Elizabeth Abinsay. "Serving the medical needs of our fellow immigrants is both fulfilling and gratifying."

A Collaborative Effort

BCWW is a continuing collaborative endeavor with the Hawai'i State Department of Health Lanakila Easy Access Program (LEAP). Services provided by BCWW volunteers serve as stop-gap measures to help newly-arrived immigrants and migrants requiring immediate medical and dental attention. Screenings and referrals are carried out of the LEAP Office of Bilingual Health Services whose staff assists in completing assessment and coordinating referrals based on the specialty, location and work schedule of the volunteer health care provider.

"These free medical services are designed to supplement, not replicate, other state and private health care agencies providing services to low-income and indigent families," says Dr. Arnold Villafuerte, LEAP Coordinator. "Moreover, by virtue of their basic remedial nature, such services should not be considered alternative health care clinics for immigrants," he added.

Funding Source

Like any non-profit organization that provides free services, funding is always an issue. The organization's answer to this problem is to form Doctors-on-Stage, an all-amateur unpaid group of performers showcasing the artistic talents of the physician volunteers, their family members, friends and office staff. Under the leadership of long-time producer Dr.Sonido, the group has staged 4 major musical productions since 2000 – "In Tune with War and Peace", "The Rainbow Connection", "Butterflies & Kisses: It Takes a Village to Raise a Child" and "Love Stories: Love Never Dies" - to raise funds through corporate and individual sponsorships and ticket sales.

In the past the State of Hawai'i Department of Health, through its Immigrant Health Initiative Program, partly supported BCWW but unfortunately state budgeting for this program has been cut as of October 1, 2009.

An Ongoing Project

Bayanihan Clinic Without Walls embodies the deep commitment, dedication, teamwork and spirit of volunteerism of a group of professionals who care enough to help the less fortunate members of the community as our expression of the Aloha spirit.

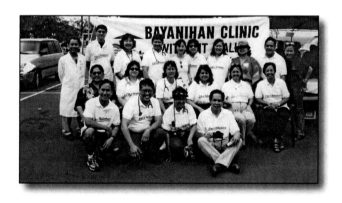

To learn more about the organization please visit www. bayanihanclinicwwhawaii.org. For further inquiries or for tax-deductible donations please write to:

The Secretariat
94-837 Waipahu St
Waipahu, HI 96797
Tel. 808-671-3911
Fax. 808-677-2720

Aloha, the Message of Hawai'i to the World

Constantine Ikaika Nightingdale

"Ua mau ke ea o ka aina i ka pono" *"The life of the land is perpetuated in righteousness."*

- Hawai'i State Emblem

Hawai'i State Flower - Hibiscus

Hawai'i State Bird - Nene Goose

Hawai'i is best known for Diamond Head, Waikiki, Volcanos & Surfing

One way to better experience this rich culture and to keep the "Aloha Spirit" alive throughout the world as a message of ALOHA is by learning a little of the Hawaiian language.

Hawaiian is a very old language which belongs to the Polynesian language family. It is closely related to other Polynesian languages which are spread over a large area of the Pacific Ocean like Micronesia, Polynesia, Melanesia, etc. Generally speaking, it appears that foreign Tahitians (some scholars estimate) colonized the Hawaiian Islands around AD 1000.

Hawai'i is the only state in the U.S.A. to have two languages – Hawaiian and English. There is a third language which is widely spoken in Hawai'i commonly called Pidgin or Hawaiian slang. Visiting Hawai'i for the first time, you will not be able to understand the pidgin or Hawaiian slang, however, once you live in Hawai'i for awhile you will catch on to pidgin & the Hawaiian slang gestures.

When Captain Cook first arrived in the Hawaiian Islands in 1778, he discovered that the Hawaiians had no written language. In 1820, missionaries began to develop and standardize a written version of the Hawaiian language. The Hawaiian language consists of only 12 letters. Seven consonants - h, k, l, m, n, p and w, and five vowels - a, e, i, o and u.

The "w" when followed by an "i" or "e" is pronounced like a "v". The vowels are a little different in that each one is pronounced individually and sound like:

a sounds like "ah" as in hurrah

e sounds like "ay" as in day

i sounds like "ee" as in bee

o sounds like "o" as in role

u sounds like "oo" as in soon

"Aloha," in my estimation, is the most used Hawaiian word in Hawai'i & around the world. In the Hawaiian language, it can mean hello, goodbye, love, welcome, affection , compassion, mercy, sympathy, pity, kindness, grace, charity; greeting, salutation, regards; sweetheart, lover, loved one; beloved, loving, kind, compassionate, charitable, lovable; to love, be fond of; to show kindness, mercy, pity, charity, affection; to venerate; to remember with affection and to greet.

The word aloha is used in a combination with other words, like aloha auinala used as a greeting that means good afternoon. Hawai'i is called the Aloha State because of our Aloha spirit and hospitality. Often I will address people when I answer the phone with aloha or when I call someone, I will greet them with Aloha then their first name. Even with my emails, I address people with Aloha & finish off with Mahalo Nui Loa (thank you very much).

The History and Formation of the State of Hawai'i

The islands were united under a single ruler, Kamehameha I, for the first time in 1810 with the help of

U.S.A. weapons and U.S.A. business men. The Hawaiian kingdom then adopted a flag similar to the one used today by the State of Hawai'i.

Prince Liholiho in May 1819 became King Kamehameha II. By his stepmother, Kalahumanu, he had abolished the kapu system that had ruled life in Hawai'i for many generations. King Kamehameha II sat down to eat with Kalahumanu and other women of chiefly rank. This act was forbidden under the old King Kamehameha I system during his time.

George Paulet, on February 10, 1843, on the Navy warship HMS Carysfort entered Honolulu and demanded that King Kamehameha III cede the Hawaiian Islands to the British Crown. Kamehameha III stepped down under military type protest.

Admiral Richard Darton Thomas arrived at Honolulu harbor on July 26, 1843. Thomas repudiated Paulet's actions, and on July 1843, restored the Hawaiian government. In his restoration speech, Kamehameha III declared that "Ua mau ke ea o ka āina i ka pono", the motto of the future State of Hawai'i translated as "The life of the land is perpetuated in righteousness." This saying is on Hawai'i's State Emblem today and can be found at the Hawai'i State Capitol and on the Hawai'i State website.

In 1875 the Kingdom of Hawai'i and the United States allowed for importation of Hawaiian sugar into the United States beginning in 1876. In exchange, Hawai'i ceded Pearl Harbor and aligning areas, free of cost to the U.S.A. This treaty acknowledged Hawai'i as a sovereign nation.

The 1887 Caucasians stripped the monarchy of much of its authority, imposed significant income and requirements for voting, and dismantled all Asians from voting. Kalākaua died in 1891. His sister Lililuokalani took over the throne.

A plot by Princess Lililuokalani was exposed to overthrow King David Kalākaua in a military up-rise in 1888. In 1889, a rebellion of Native Hawaiians attempted to replace the unpopular Bayonet Constitution and stormed Iolani Palace. The take-over was crushed by the U.S.A. Marines in January 1893. Queen Lililuokalani, immediately upon ascending the throne received petitions from two-thirds of her subjects and the major Native Hawaiian political party, asking her to proclaim a new constitution. Lililuokalani drafted a new constitution that would restore the monarchy's authority. Due to Lililuokalani's suspected actions, a group of Americans and Europeans formed a Committee on January 14, 1893. The Committee committed itself to removing the Queen and annexation to the United States. United States Government Minister Mr. Stevens summoned a company of uniformed USA Marines from the USS Boston and companies of US sailors to land and take up positions at the USA Consulate. In January 16, 1893 the Committee had claimed an imminent threat to the American lives. The Provisional Government of Hawai'i was established to manage the Hawaiian people. Queen Lililuokalani left her throne. The Queen's statement yielding the Hawaiian Kingdom happened on January 17, 1893.

A joint resolution was written by Congressman Newlands to annex Hawai'i. McKinley signed the Newlands Resolution which officially annexed Hawai'i on July 1898 to become the Territory of Hawai'i. On February 1900 a territorial government was established with a governor appointed by the US President. The territorial legislature convened for the first time in February 1901.

President Dwight D. Eisenhower signed the Hawai'i Admission Act on 1959 which allowed for Hawaiian statehood. Hawai'i was admitted as the 50th state on August 1959.

Hawai'i is well known for its splendid climate, great beaches and beautiful scenery. Once you arrive in Hawai'i, you find that it is much more. You find an inviting and rich culture much different than the one you may experience on the mainland & fresh air compared to Los Angeles. While the Hawaiian language was once almost dead, in recent years the Hawaiian language has been making a comeback.

Clothing, Dance and Food as part of the Hawaiian Culture

While day dreaming about your Hawai'i trip, visions of women in grass skirts adorning your neck with a beautiful lei upon your arrival at the airport have undoubtedly crossed your mind. Unfortunately, unless you are meeting a family member, friend, or someone that wants to greet you the Hawaiian way with a lei, you will not get one.

The Aloha shirt goes back to the time of the 19th century when the early Western missionaries took notice of the need to have the natives be properly clothed in preparation for their conversion to Christianity. The shirts had flamboyant colors and tropical prints. It wasn't until the 1930's that the aloha shirt went into commercial production. A Honolulu Chinese merchant by the name of Mr. Chun and owner of King-Smith Clothiers, was believed to be the pioneer of the Aloha Shirt. Along with his sister, Ethel Chun, they manufactured the first vibrantly colored, floral shirts from left-over Japanese kimono fabric.

Hawai'i's Luaus are a great way for you to experience Hawaiian dancing, culture & food. Hawai'i Luaus are traditional ways to celebrate graduations, weddings, baby's arrivals and birthdays. Most of the time, Hawai'i Luaus are held in the backyard under tents, parks or at beaches. Throughout the Mainland US, you can taste some of Hawai'i's food by visiting L & L Barbeque, a franchise that started in Hawai'i with a local type menu.

The Ohana (family) Values, Hawai'i's Communities, Health & Wellness sets Hawai'i above and as a leader the U.S.A. in health & living longer. A healthy Hawai'i and healthy community are general ideas for getting out and exercising and enjoying the outdoors. In certain places in the U.S.A. and around the world snow would hinder people from going out on cold days, however, with Hawai'i there are no cold days. The people of Hawai'i are able to enjoy year around sun and recreation.

Hawai'i's Present Challenges

Today, our paradise is in a crisis with many problems - The Hawaiian Islands have approximately 26,000 to 28,000 homeless with 10,000 homeless alone on the Island of Oahu. Hawai'i also has a population of over 4,000 to 6,000 men and women that are incarcerated. Due to the high costs and prison overcrowding, approximately 2,000 of Hawai'i's imprisoned men have been moved to Arizona. Also, there are nearly 8,000 to 10,000 men and women that are on probation and approximately 4,000 children whose parents are in prison.

Hawai'i has 100 active gangs that have an overall total of 4,000 to 6,000 gang members (gang markings are in almost every community in Hawai'i with graffiti & shoes hanging from telephone wires). Every month, one woman dies due to domestic violence and at least one person commits suicide. Hawai'i is rated 5th in the US for the drug use of Methamphetamine, also simply known as Meth. Hawai'i was once #1 for Meth use.

With this said, Hawai'i is still one of the most beautiful places to visit and live. This is why so many people are moving to Hawai'i from the mainland, Korea, China, Japan, Micronesia, Samoa, Tonga, & other places. Our vision for a better Hawai'i is by "Changing Hawai'i's Communities for the better now in order to create a brighter future for tomorrow." In order to improve Hawai'i's quality of life, Hawai'i must first set its priority to instill hope in the people of Hawai'i by guiding them to live healthy and productive lives. We must look at all the aspects of life in Hawai'i such as government, schools, transportation, self sustainability, spiritual aspects, working climates, sovereignty, accountability, economy, cultures, our history, family values, communities, health, & wellness. It is only by working in a true relationship of OHANA will we ever send "ALOHA," The Message of Hawai'i to the World.

****

Mr. Constantine I. Nightingdale, President & CEO, Hawai'i Dream Service Center (HDSC) www.hawaiidreamservice. org & Chairman, Hawai'i Christian Community Foundation (HPCCF) & Chairman, Hawai'i Community Land Trust (HCLT). Mr. Constantine Nightingdale has served as the Island of Oahu Community Volunteer Legal Services Program, as the Island wide legal advocate for local attorneys with varied legal services To Build A Better Hawai'i - Changing Hawai'i's Communities For The Better now in order to create a brighter future for tomorrow. He has also served as the Hawaiian Islands Director for Chuck Colsen's Angel Tree Network on the islands of Oahu, Maui, Kauai, Lanai, Molokai, & the Big Island, networking with hundreds of local churches and working with thirty-five hundred children of incarcerated parents island wide. For the past 12 years he has served as an island wide social net-worker and community builder.

He has held community outreach events in Waianae on the island of Oahu for over 1,000 people and in Waipahu for over 500 people. He has served as the Assistant Administrator of the second largest nursing facility in Hawai'i in charge of five departments and responsible for accounting, finance, contract negotiation, vendor services, marketing, hiring, scheduling, supervision, and customer service administration. He has also served as an assistant professor at the University of Hawai'i. He has held community events at the Ala Moana Hotel and Pacific Beach Hotel for hundreds local churches and hundreds of local non-profits and community leaders. He helped develop Veterans Program in Barbers Point & seven other nonprofits with responsibility of financial modeling, gross margin improvement, revenue forecasting & expansion, strategic pricing & planning, funding, profit & loss reporting & facility development. He has assisted in numerous island-wide prayer events with thousands in attendance.

He has a degree from the UH, CIA, US Navy A & C schools and other certificates. As an instructor for the US Navy, Mr. Nightingdale holds the "Master Training Specialist", the Navy's highest training award. He served in the US Navy with 9 flagstaffs, USS Carl Vincent, USS Gridley, RTC-NTC San-Diego, Navy Base Long Beach, and others. He has owned dozens of businesses and networks with Community & Christian organizations, churches, ministries & has launched dozens of entrepreneurship businesses. He has appeared on TBN TV, LeSea TV, OLELO TV, Akaka-Maui Community TV, Ho'ike-Kauai Community TV, Na Leo TV, KGMB TV, KFVE TV, KHNK TV, KHON2 TV, KITV & Salem Broadcasting and has had a local community show on all the Hawaiian Islands. He has written numerous articles on homeless, gangs, human trafficking and other social issues relating to Hawai'i's Past, Present & Future. He is 52 years old, married with 3 children and attends New Hope Christian Fellowship with his family for over 12 years.

Mr. Constantine I. Nightingdale
President/CEO
HAWAII DREAM SERVICE CENTER
1312 Arsenal Rd.
Honolulu, Hawaii 96819
Main Office: (808) 285-3622
Administrative Office: (808) 853-2025
Website: www.hawaiidreamservicecenter.org
Email: cnightingdale@yahoo.com

`A`ohe hana nui ke alu `ia

No task is too big when done together by all.

Now What Is Next?

Together with Aloha, WE Can Make A Difference

"Aloha, The Message of Hawai'i" not only shares the deeper meaning of this valuable part of the culture of Hawai'i, but also comes with a clear mission to help preserve the spirit of Aloha in the islands, maintain the best quality of life for the people, celebrate the natural God-given gifts and talents of the islands' youth, provide more dignity and opportunity to those less fortunate, and share with the world the love and harmony that comes from Aloha. We hope you will join us in carrying out this mission.

This is not the end, but just the beginning. *Each* of our islands' brothers, sisters, cousins, and even the guests we gladly welcome to visit, who share with us this beautiful and blessed land, *is important* and has something good to contribute. Our shared piece of paradise can continue

133

to be the way we know it if each one of us, regardless of age or background, commits to do his/her part to help preserve "the spirit of Aloha" in our land.

While I was writing this last chapter, I learned about the world renowned singer and Hawaiians' beloved musical artist Israel "IZ" Kamakawiwo'ole. I couldn't stop listening to his beautiful rendition of two of my most favorite songs – *Somewhere Over the Rainbow* and *What a Wonderful World*. His official website commented, "Music was his passion; his family and friends were his treasure." Remember those songs that lift your hearts and spirits, as if listening to "IZ," the Hawaiian Suppaman when he said, *"Facing future I see hope, hope that we will survive, hope that we will prosper, hope that once again we will reap the blessings of this magical land, for without hope I cannot live; remember the past but not dwell there, face the future where all our hopes stand."* Brudda Iz, as he was fondly called, will always be remembered as the singer with the small ukulele and a huge heart filled with Aloha. Search his name on the Internet to hear more of IZ's story and his Aloha-filled songs which are bound to live forever.

Never lose HOPE, as the rainbows never cease to appear over our islands. Never lose sight of what makes Hawai'i a very special home for us, and a delightful place for many who come to visit and discover the essence that surrounds these paradise islands of ours. IT

IS THE ALOHA, the never-to-fade message of love and harmony among the people of Hawai'i, willingly being shared with the world.

Many different groups, associations or organizations may have different causes or functions, and yet can still come together as a larger community to share this simple common goal that can only benefit us all. Gladly working, sharing with one another, and caring for each other - are traits that make Aloha what it is all about. Together, we can do it. Together, with the same heart and spirit of Aloha, we can continue to see good things happen. We can keep this land and each of us HAPPY and HEALTHY, the ALOHA way.

Mahalo! May God bless you and us all.

Just as I finalized the manuscript of this book and was preparing for the next phase, news about the tremendous earthquake and tsunami that hit Japan was all over. On Friday, March 11, 2011, according to the news, the biggest earthquake to hit Japan in 140 years struck the northeast coast. At a record 8.9 magnitude, it triggered a 10-meter tsunami that uprooted trees and swept away houses, buildings, cars, boats and everything else in its path. All was washed away or destroyed in just a matter of hours, yet the impact and memory of this moment to the Japanese people, and even to the rest of the world, will surely last for a very long time. Ten of thousands were presumed dead. Thousands more were injured or scattered among temporary shelters as they lost their homes or properties. Then, the fear of the possible meltdown of some of Japan's nuclear reactors and the spread of radiation engulfed people.

Most of the world seemed to pause as TV footage showed the stunning devastation of Japan's calamities. The thought of the potential effect of what was happening to Japan weighed on neighboring nations and everyone else around the globe. Offers of help from everywhere poured in. Then, somehow, people watching the news on television or the internet began to notice *something special*, beyond the effect of powerful natural disasters that can hit anyone anytime. It was the spirit of Aloha coming alive across the globe! This can be best described by actual comments posted on blogs from around the world. Here were few:

Japan your broken hearts are felt around the world. – B

I just have to think of this when I think I'm having a bad day and it doesn't even matter after that. God Bless the Japanese people and help them through this horrific crisis. – Mr. CI

Unfortunately it is in times like these that we should remind ourselves to be thankful and not take for granted the things we have in this life because it can be gone in a blink of an eye. Japan has a long and hard road to recovery. So today before you start to complain, or whine about this or that or about anything petty, look no further than your TV screen and the horrific scenes on the news to remind yourself that you have it pretty good. Keep Japan in your prayers. - Ms M

The Japanese students in the shelters have been great, helping with the cooking and cleaning up, caring for the elderly, bringing water. – R

I can't believe my eyes, very few if any negative posts. This is the way people should be, helping our fellow man not dishing out hate. So let's take a lesson from the country of Japan and her people. Respect and love for your fellow man though they may look different, talk different, and do things in a different way. We are all together on this small planet so let us act in a loving and kind way to each other. I pray that the people of Japan can pull out of this with heads held high. – Mr. Y

May God bless the people of Japan and the land of the rising sun. Many share your loss and are praying for your healing and speedy recovery.

Japan's despair and devastation, and facing the challenge of feeding and housing hundreds of thousands of homeless survivors, at the same time brought awareness, realization, reflection, and life lessons to humankind. It brought a realization that life is too short, and you never know when your life here on earth will suddenly end. How do you live your life? Are you living in fear, stress or anxiety, or do you have the peace and hope to carry on? What other good lessons can be learned?

Something definitely has changed for many people around the globe who have been touched by Japan's disasters. I developed friendships with some Japanese Americans here in Hawai'i, and some of them are actually contributors to this book project. Their ways of life impressed me as a reflection of Aloha. These beautiful friends and newly adopted families, together with their fellow countrymen have made a lasting impact on the lives of people everywhere. Thank you for sharing with us your grace, strength and integrity in dealing with life, others, and such tremendous crisis. Mahalo for being a great example for us to learn from.

Yes, I learned so much in the last few days, weeks and months, -far more than in my many years of school and career learning. I learned more about life, the earth, the forces of the universe, and the nature of human beings. Personally, these are the more valuable lessons in life that helped me define the reason for my existence, my purpose and what I have to do for my remaining days as God wills it. The message of Aloha brought more meaning to my life, and for sure will guide me to carry on. Each life is a story. Each of us is creating one.

"Aloha, The Message of Hawai'i" has found its ultimate purpose: to spread the message of Aloha throughout the world. Aloha does not have to be confined to the islands of Hawai'i alone. While we make every effort to preserve the spirit of Aloha in Hawai'i, this valuable part of our culture can be lovingly shared with others, anywhere and everywhere, who are open and willing to adapt to something beautiful and meaningful. Imagine living in a world where you consider everyone to be your dear cousins, good neighbors, great friends or extended family you can always count on. We welcome and care for each other, and we are always ready to extend a helping hand, to share and support one another. I for one still have so much to learn and practice.

I have a dream, and perhaps it is just a dream. But I have made up my mind that it is better for me to hold on to that dream than to brush it off and do nothing about it. I feel I can share this with you because I know I am not alone in my dream: More than ever, people around the globe will gather to share among themselves the true meaning of health and wellness. It is not all just physically or financially focused, but involves integrated areas including spiritual, mental, emotional and social for TOTAL WELLNESS so we can truly enjoy

ABUNDANCE in all aspects of life, and learn how to attain it individually and collectively.

We learn how awakening ourselves to the TRUTH can actually bring healing to our entire being. We learn how, if we govern ourselves with simple, uncomplicated, unconditional LOVE, we can achieve VICTORY.

One can only wonder why there are conflicts and wars, as results of selfishness, greed, control or power hunger, when it is so much easier and less costly to simply love and care, and be always willing to give and share. Only true love wins. It's only LOVE that conquers all. True love only comes from God. The essence and spirit of ALOHA is what we need.

The only question is, can we still see, hear and learn?

Thinking of the whole galaxy, we are to realize that Earth is a small world after all.

In closing, without being religious, as religions are but manmade, please allow me to quote a few well-known or favorite verses that have more authority than my words alone. These may bring more sense to what's truly going on as we ponder their meaning:

"And you shall know the truth, and the truth shall make you free."

John 8:32

"The thief does not come except to steal, and to kill, and to destroy. I have come that they may have life, and that they may have it more abundantly."

John 10:10

"For God so loved the world that He gave His only begotten Son, that whoever believes in Him should not perish but have everlasting life."

John 3:16

And then there is, I Corinthians 13, the Love Chapter:

Though I speak with the tongues of men and of angels, but have not love, I have become sounding brass or a clanging cymbal. And though I have the gift of prophecy, and understand all mysteries and all knowledge, and though I have all faith, so that I could remove mountains, but have not love, I am nothing. And though I bestow all my goods to feed the poor, and though I give my body to be burned, but have not love, it profits me nothing.

Love suffers long and is kind; love does not envy; love does not parade itself, is not puffed up; does not behave rudely, does not seek its own, is not provoked, thinks no evil; does not rejoice in iniquity, but rejoices in the truth; bears all things, believes all things, hopes all things, endures all things. Love never fails. But whether there are prophecies, they will fail;

whether there are tongues, they will cease; whether there is knowledge, it will vanish away. For we know in part and we prophesy in part. But when that which is perfect has come, then that which is in part will be done away.

When I was a child, I spoke as a child, I understood as a child, I thought as a child; but when I became a man, I put away childish things. For now we see in a mirror, dimly, but then face to face. Now I know in part, but then I shall know just as I also am known. And now abide faith, hope, love, these three; but the greatest of these is love.

Hawaiians are blessed with Aloha! In turn, "Aloha" is Hawai'i's beautiful gift to the world, to humanity. Aloha is an expression of a warm or affectionate greetings, love, compassion or caring. It is a good practice to exercise Aloha every moment of the day. It brings wellness to your soul, mind and body. Together, let's share our Aloha spirit and make the world a better place. Together, WE can make a difference. Mahalo!

To you, as always with all our hearts,

Aloha!

****

Recommended websites to find out more about Aloha and Hawai'i:

www.gohawaii.com
www.AlohaClubHawaii.com

"What do you like/love about Hawai'i?"
"What does Aloha mean to you?"

When our Locals, Visitors and Guests were asked these questions, here are their answers:

"What does aloha mean to us?

Although grammatically "aloha" means welcome, hello or goodbye, the word really means much more than those greetings. The word aloha itself identifies Hawaii and all its islands and to my family it is a feeling of second home, vacation, recreation, leisure, beautiful warm ocean, beautiful birds, sight and smell of beautiful flowers, leis, hula dance, music, picnics, barbecues and luaus. Aloha is truly Hawaiian, and for those who have visited and experienced Hawaii, the word aloha gives one a feeling of everyday vacation and a sense of an earthly paradise. This is a special place on earth that seems calling you to come back, and that you would love to keep going back to. It must be the spirit of Aloha!"

– Virgil & June Romeroso
Entrepreneurs
Silicon Valley, California

"What Aloha means to me: Aloha is the spirit of togetherness and warmth from those around you and even the strangers you meet with an instant expression of love. Aloha can also build strength in relationships and develop the Ohana into a tight knit bond that will never break."

– Nathan McCotter
Entrepreneur
Honolulu, Hawaii

"What we both love about Hawaii is not only the breathtaking beauty of the beaches, plants and flowers, fruit plantations, mountains and hills, and other aspects of its natural scenery, or the rich and fascinating history of the culture and how it was preserved and passed on through the generations through the music, dancing and folklore, but also – and above everything else – we simply love the warmth and hospitality of the people. Everyone that we meet is so welcoming and loving. For us, that is "Aloha": that spirit of warmth and love passed on through the ages and extended not only to family and friends, but to virtually everyone who crosses their path."

– Alex & Pauline Cabansagan
Pastor & Freelance Journalist
Daly City/San Francisco, CA.

"Business the 'Aloha' way - I love the sense of, and the importance placed on "Ohana." Clients are not dollar signs, but someone's mom, father, child, sister, brother, etc., and everyone has unique situations and problems. Aloha is about remembering the individual and maintaining respect. Aloha is about human connection and not the corporate, machine-like treatment of people. Aloha is about sincerity, honesty and continual commitment to achieving results regardless of the time and effort required. To preserve Aloha, we must treat all clients the same, regardless of income, credit, loan size or situation. Every individual is important; it's our job to make them know this when they walk out our doors."

– Maria Williams
Entrepreneur
Kapolei, Hawaii

"Malama (caring) and Kuleana (responsible). These Hawaiian words – the human essence of those words –

have paved the way to pure Aloha in my life. First, I want to be Malama to myself and to others, and with all I do. Then, I want to be Kuleana for all my life's experiences and emotions. With that journey taking place, I am able to truly experience the Aloha that Hawaii is known for. Aloha for ourselves, Aloha for other human beings, Aloha for the world we live in."

– Eli Zollo
Accountant
Kaneohe, Hawaii

"Upon arrival in Hawaii, I immediately get captivated by the smile of the people. Hawaii speaks to me of love and warmth."

– Claire Melvilee
San Jose, California

"What Aloha means to me?

Ten years ago, my brother and I shared many thoughts and dreams while living in the Philippines. We went to the rooftop and watched those diamond-like stars up in the sky while dreaming of living in a foreign land. I was 14 years old then. In 2005, part of my family came to Hawaii. The first thing I heard from the people in the airport was a loud A-l-o-h-a! I had mixed emotions. I was happy knowing we've finally reuniting with our relatives. I was sad, lonely and teary that my two brothers didn't come with us to this new country. I was angry that I left all my friends and could no longer hang out with them. Days passed, and the feeling of being a stranger slowly went away because of the Aloha spirit. People in Hawaii are friendly.

Everybody must be wondering why I am telling my story and what the connection is to what aloha means to me. Well, aloha is not just a word. It's not just as simple as saying 'hello' or 'hi.' Aloha means happiness, love and compassion. My family shows the spirit of it by being hospitable. We treat strangers like friends and visitors like family. We show and offer them the best of Hawaii there is. I often used this word in welcoming somebody, a greeting for a brand new day. I've also used it just to ask for some attention. The power of aloha can actually give a positive outcome to something or positive attitude to people that can improve one's life.

Every time I hear this greeting I think of my brothers, wishing they were here with us, hoping that one day they will be joining us at a luau. A luau is a gathering serving the best of Hawaiian foods and entertainment. The spirit of aloha cannot only be felt by saying the word itself, it is more about applying the meaning into action. For me, it has more meaning - a deeper meaning. Aloha means family, friendship, and now it means a home."

– Roxan Bantolina
Medical Assistant
Aiea, Hawaii

(A postcard picked up at the reception table of Hawai'i Visitors & Convention Bureau titled "Live Aloha" bears this message by an anonymous writer...)

"ALOHA... the embodiment of the essence of Hawai'i! To the people of the islands, Aloha is more than a word of greeting, farewell or salutation... it's a way of life. Aloha means mutual regard and affection and extends warmth in caring with no expectation of anything in return.

Regardless of where we live, we are all part of a global community, and our connection to one another is based on mutual respect for our differences as well as our appreciation for what we have in common.

Community is the sum of individuals – individuals who have concern for one another, who care, share and take responsibility.

Aloha is a gift to be shared, and it is up to each of us to be stewards of this gift. To share Aloha, we must each make a commitment to live in a manner that expresses Aloha to all we come into contact with each day, and to undertake a set of actions that demonstrate the Spirit of Aloha."

– Live Aloha
www.ealoha.com/livaloha.htm

Hawaiian Proverbs, Favorite Quotes and Phrases

Ua Mau ke Ea o ka 'Äina i ka Pono
The life of the land is perpetuated by righteousness.
- State Motto

Malama Kekahi i kekahi
Take care of each other.
- Hawaiian Proverb

Nana ka maka, hana ka lima
Watch and you will learn how to do it.
- Hawaiian Proverb

`A`ohe hana nui ke alu `ia
No task is too big when done together by all.
- Hawaiian Proverb

Pupukahi i holomua
Unite in order to progress.
- Hawaiian Proverb

'A'ohe lokomaika'i i nele i ke pān'i
No kind deed has ever lacked its reward.
An opportunity to help another is a gift. To live with Aloha is
to have a giving nature.
Give for the pleasure of giving. Do not expect something in
return.

E lawe i ke a`o a malama, a e `oi mau ka na`auao
He who takes his teachings and applies them increases his
knowledge.

Ho'omoe wai kāhi ke kāo'o
Let us all travel together like water flowing in one direction
Live in harmony with other people and the world around you.

I ulu no ka lala i ke kumu
The reach of a tree's branches depends on its trunk
A family's unconditional love strengthens each one to succeed.

Ua ola loko i ke aloha
Love gives life within.

He kēhau ho'oma'ema'e ka aloha
Love is like a cleansing dew.
The cleansing power of Aloha can soothe and heal.
Love removes hurt. Love conquers all.

Pa`a ka waha
Observe, be silent and learn.
If words are exiting your mouth, wisdom cannot come in

I la maika'i nou
Have a nice day!

Aloha ke Ahua...
God is Love.
- Daniel Kaniela Akaka, Jr.

As the Hawaiians say, *Hele me kahau 'oli* -- go with joy.
- Gilbert M. Grosvenor

Hawaii has the key and that key is ALOHA.
- Pilahi Paki

The meaning of Aloha comes from the heart and is given freely.

The spiritual meaning to each letter of the word aloha:

A stands for AKAHAI, meaning kindness, expressed with tenderness.

L is for LOKAHI, meaning unity, expressed with harmony.

O is for OLU`OLU, meaning agreeable, expressed with pleasantness.

H stands for HA`AHA`A, meaning humility, expressed with modesty.

A stands for AHONUI, meaning patient and persevering.

Written by Hawaiian poet and philosopher Pilahi Paki, a renowned and beloved linguist. Adopted by the Hawaii Legislature in 1986 ([§5-7.5] Aloha Spirit)

I believe Hawaii is the most precious jewel in the world.
- Don Ho

Aloha is the unconditional desire to promote the true good of other people in a friendly spirit out of a sense of kinship.
- Abraham Akaka

Nature is where it all begins for the Hawaiians. In fact, they call themselves keiki o ka 'aina-- 'children of the land'.
- M.J. Harden

Hawaii is paradise born of fire.
- Rand McNally

I thought my book was done, then we went to Hawaii and the whole last chapter happened.
- Mariel Hemingway

When you're there at sunset or when you see the moonlight on the water, Waikiki is just unbeatable.
- Rick Egged

Hawaii is the land of big dreams, for both islanders and guests. Those dreams born in Paradise can, indeed, come true.
- Sharon Linnea

The aloha spirit and the concept of ohana are not mere words to us, they mean that we care for each other including those we don't know.
– Linda Lingle

All Hawaii beaches are open to the public - there's no such thing as a private beach.
- Neil Abercrombie

Hula is the language of the heart and therefore the heartbeat of the Hawaiian people.
- David (Kâwika) La'amea Kalâkaua, King of Hawaii, 1874 to 1891

Hula is the art of Hawaiian dance, which expresses all we see, smell, taste, touch, feel, and experience. It is joy, sorrow, courage, and fear.

- Robert Cazimero

The hands of the hula dancer are ever going out in gesture, her body swaying and pivoting itself in attitude of expression. Her whole physique is a living and moving picture of feeling, sentiment, and passion.

- Nathaniel B. Emerson

One 'ukulele and one soul can do a lot.

- Kindy Sproat

If we lose this thing called "aloha," we're just like any sand-and-surf destination. I don't believe we can afford to go there.

— Rex Johnson

Hawaii has the ability to bring people together in an environment of trust, positive energy, and warmth. Within this environment interactions occur that catalyze the beginnings of great things.

- Burt Lum, Honolulu Advertiser

The key to life is to live ALOHA everyday!

- AlohaClubHawaii.com

Wherever you go, God be with you.

– Israel "IZ" Kamakawiwo'Ole

Aloha, never leave home without it.

– Jon de Mello

We hope you will embrace the spirit of aloha in your everyday lives; for it is not a gift only for those who visit Hawaii, it is a gift which can be shared throughout the world.

– University of Hawaii Community Colleges website: uhcc. Hawaii.edu/aloha/alohaSpirit.php

Live Aloha

Respect all elders and children.
Leave places better than you find them.
Hold the door. Hold the elevator.
Plant something.
Drive with courtesy. Never drive impaired.
Attend an event of another culture.
Return your shopping cart.
Get out and enjoy nature.
Pick up litter.
Share with your neighbors.
Create smiles.
Create a list and share it.

You don't have to be a politician,
Or the president of a company.
Or a famous doctor,
To make everyone's life better.
Sometimes the smallest things make
the biggest difference.

The sharing of Aloha comes from the heart... shared from person to person.
And to Live Aloha we should consider the guiding words of Queen Lili'uokalani:
Let only the golden blossoms of aloha live in your heart...

Let us all Live Aloha... Now more than ever!!!
- Live Aloha ealoha.com/livaloha.htm

Glossary of Most Common Hawaiian Terms:

Aloha – Welcome, Hello, Goodbye, Love

Aloha kakahiaka - Good morning

Aloha `auinala - Good afternoooon

Aloha Au Ia 'Oe - I Love You

Aloha Aku No, Aloha Mai No - I give my love to you, you give your love to me

Aloha No Au Ia 'Oe - I Truly Love You

Kai - The Sea

Kamaaina - Native-born (kama: child; of the aina: land)

Kamaaina Kipa hou mai - Come visit again

Kane - Man

Keiki - Child or Children, Baby

Mahalo – Thank you

Mahalo nui loa - Thank you very much

Mahalo E Ke Akua No Keia La - Thanks be to God for this day

Nau ko`u aloha - My love is yours

Ohana - Family

Wahine - Woman

Wahi noho like o ka po'e – Community

Other Terms:

Akamai - Smart

Aloha `oe - Farewell to you

Aloha Kakou - May there be love between us (said to more than one person)

'Ao'ao – Directions

Kuleana –Responsibility

Malama – Care, caring

Male Ana E Pili Mai Aloha Kaua - We two will cling to love in marriage

Me Ke Aloha Pumehana - With the warmth of my love

No Keia La, No Keia Po, A Mau Loa - From this day, from this night, forever more

Special Occasions:

Ho`olaule`a - Celebration

Palapala kono - Invitation

Manawa - Date/Time

Kauwahi - Place

Hau`oli la Hanau - Happy Birthday

Ho'omaika'i 'ana - Congratulations

Hau`oli la Ho'omana'o - Happy Anniversary

Hau`oli la Ho'omaha loa - Happy Retirement

Hau'oli Makahiki Hou - Happy New Years

Ho'omaha loa - Retirement/Retire

Ko maua la male 'ana - Our Wedding Day

La hanau – Birthday

Male 'ana - Wedding

Mele Kalikimaka - Merry Christmas

Days of the Week:

Lapule - Sunday

Po'akahi - Monday

Po'alua - Tuesday

Po'akolu - Wednesday

Po'aha - Thursday

Po'alima - Friday

Po 'aono - Saturday

Months:

'Iaunuali - January

Pepeluali - February

Malaki - March

'Apelila - April

Mei - May

Iune - June

Iulai - July

'Aukake - August

Kepakemapa - September

'Okakopa - October

Nowemapa - November

Kekemapa - December

Numbers:

'Ekahi - One

'Elua - Two

'Ekolu - Three

'Eha - Four

'Elima - Five

'Eono - Six

'Ehiku - Seven

'Ewalu - Eight

'Eiwa - Nine

'Umi - Ten

The Islands of Hawai'i

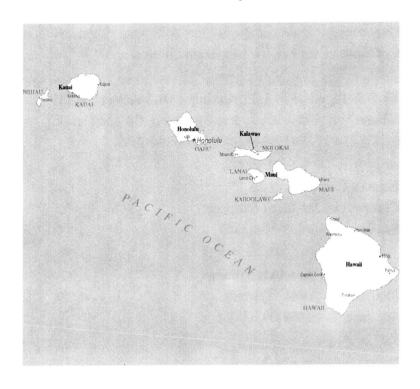

Special Acknowledgement

Our deepest appreciation to the following Sponsors and Contributors for helping us make a difference.

VLF & Together MAD (Making A Difference) TEAM
Silicon Valley/Bay Area - San Francisco, CA and Hawai'i
(408)871-0377/(415)424-9801/(808)294-4499

Hassan Company
Commercial Janitorial Services
San Jose, CA (408)358-3303

Sam Russell/AccelAir Systems
Mechanical, HVAC Systems
San Jose, CA (408)282-1180

Smart Solutions 24-7
Administrative Virtual Assistance Services
Honolulu, HI (808)294-4499

CPSIA information can be obtained at www.ICGtesting.com
Printed in the USA
238386LV00005B/79/P